yellow fever

A DEADLY DISEASE POISED TO KILL AGAIN

yellow fever

james l. dickerson

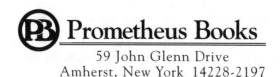

Prometheus Books

59 John Glenn Drive
Amherst, New York 14228-2197

Library of Congress Cataloging-in-Publication Data

Dickerson, James.
     Yellow fever : a deadly disease poised to kill again / by James L. Dickerson.
        p. cm.
     Includes bibliographical references and index.
     ISBN 1-59102-399-8 (hardcover : alk. paper)
     1. Yellow fever—History. I. Title.
RA644.Y4.D53 2006
614.5′41—dc22

                                                                    2005038055

Printed in the United States of America on acid-free paper

To Alex A. Alston Jr.

contents

Acknowledgments   11

CHAPTER ONE

Philadelphia: The Great Plague of 1793   13

CHAPTER TWO

New Orleans: Gateway to Death   33

CHAPTER THREE

Memphis Almost Disappears   61

CHAPTER FOUR

Mississippi Devastated by Yellow Jack   103

CHAPTER FIVE

Spanish-American War: Finding the Real Enemy   141

CHAPTER SIX

    Weapons of Mass Destruction   187

CHAPTER SEVEN

    Global Warming Casts Ominous Shadow   225

CHAPTER EIGHT

    The Disease That Won't Go Away   237

Notes   253

Bibliography   261

Index   267

acknowledgments

I would like to thank the following people, institutions, and organizations for their help in writing this book: the Memphis and Shelby County Public Library, especially the staff in the Memphis and Shelby County Room; Clinton Bagley and other staff members at the Mississippi Department of Archives and History; Dr. Ned Hayes at the United States Centers for Disease Control and Prevention; Joy Victory and Margaret Neu at the *Corpus Christi Caller-Times*; Andrew L. Sallans at the Claude Moore Health Sciences Library at the University of Virginia Health System; the staff at the Flowood Public Library, Flowood, Mississippi; the staff at the Mississippi Valley Collection at the University of Memphis; the staff at the Jean and Alexander Heard Library at the Vanderbilt University Library; the staff at the William Alexander Percy Memorial Library, Greenville, Mississippi; my editor at Prometheus Books, Steven L. Mitchell, who encouraged the book's vision; and my copy editor, Jeremy Sauer, who expertly eyed the fine details.

The photos on pages 98 and 100 are courtesy the History Department of the Memphis/Shelby County Public Library and Information Center; the photos on pages 126 and 130 are courtesy of the Mississippi Department of Archives and History; and the photos on pages 158, 160, 162, 165, 166, 167, 169, 170, 171, and 176 are courtesy of the Historical Collections and Services, Claude Moore Health Sciences Library, University of Virginia.

CHAPTER ONE

philadelphia

the great plague of 1793

By 1793 Philadelphia was not the largest city in the United States—New York held that distinction by a slight margin—but with a population of 28,522, it was the second largest city and the indisputable heart and soul of the new American democracy. As the nation's first capital, Philadelphia was home to President George Washington during both of his terms, and it was the meeting place for Congress.

Spring that year followed an unusually mild winter, which had brought no snow and left the many streams that surrounded the city unencumbered with ice. The trees blossomed early, and birds filled the limbs weeks sooner than expected. Then the rains came, filling the streams and creating stagnant pools of water that resisted drainage. As a result, the city's garbage piled up along the Delaware River, creating an unbearable stench that lingered in the air and darkened the mood of those whose job it was to carry on with the business of feeding and clothing the population.

With the arrival of summer, the dampness slowly turned to drought as the streams dried up and the pastures shriveled and turned an ominous brown. Philadelphians were on edge because two years earlier a drought had contributed to fires that nearly destroyed the city. As the days wore on and the water levels of the wells dropped, there was a fear that disaster was just around the corner.

From flood to drought, the city moved toward fall with great apprehension. Flies and mosquitoes filled the stifling air, leading old-timers to warn of the dangers associated with autumnal diseases that typically followed flood-drought cycles. True enough, even as the August heat baked the city streets, yellow fever returned for the first time in over a decade, creating isolated pockets of illness all over the city.

Especially concerned was Dr. Benjamin Rush, a signer of the Declaration of Independence and the most prominent physician in the city. There was considerable disagreement among the city's physicians about the cause of the disease. Some blamed poor sanitation or the climate. Others attributed it to an influx of immigrants from Haiti and other Caribbean islands.

In mid-August, Rush was called by two physicians, Hugh Hodge and John Foulke, to the home of Peter LeMaigre, a wealthy French importer whose thirty-three-year-old wife, Catherine, was vomiting black bile and complaining of a burning heat in her stomach. Rush was unable to save the woman (she died the following day, moaning and in great pain), but he used her illness as ammunition to persuade the city that it was in the midst of a yellow fever epidemic. Philadelphians understood what that meant. Over the past one hundred years, there had been four documented yellow fever epidemics in the city, all of which had produced dire consequences.

In 1793 no one had any idea what caused yellow fever. The truth could have been found buried in an amalgamation of the theories then offered to the public—standing water, swarming insects, the arrival of ships from the Caribbean with disease-carrying "foreigners"—but at that time each possible cause had its own group of staunch defenders, and it would be more than one hundred years before the cause was pinpointed.

Just as there was a difference of opinion over the cause of yellow fever, so were there differences over how the disease should be treated. Rush's visit to the LeMaigre household is a case in point. Dr. Hodge, whose daughter already had died of yellow fever, had served as an army surgeon during the Revolutionary War. Dr. Foulke was a fellow of Philadelphia's College of Physicians and a member of the state hospital board. Hodge and Foulke gave their patient cool water spiked with apple and barley and wine laced with laudanum to help her sleep. Her face and arms were washed regularly with wet cloths.

Rush's treatment regime was considered one of the most aggressive in the city. It consisted of inducing vomiting and bowel movements with mercurial purges and bloodletting that sometimes drained up to four-fifths of the blood in the body. If his remedy did not kill the patient outright, it certainly made recovery difficult, even under the best of circumstances. The bloodletting and purges induced by Rush deprived patients of vital bodily fluids, without which there was no hope of recovery.

Rush held a unique position in Philadelphia society. He was not only one of the most respected physicians in the city (he had studied under the best surgeons in Europe) but also a political activist who had been a tireless supporter of the revolution. After the war, he contributed ideas to both federal and state constitutions. He was strongly opposed to alcohol use because he believed, correctly as it turned out, that it has an injurious effect on the stomach and liver. He also felt that alcohol affected society as a whole. Wrote Rush: "A people corrupted with strong drink cannot long be a free people. The rulers of such a community will soon partake of the vices of that mass from which they were secreted, and all our laws and governments will sooner or later bear the same marks of the effects of spirituous liquors which were described formerly upon individuals."

Rush believed that good physical and emotional health were related to good government—and vice versa. For that reason, the prospect of a serious yellow fever epidemic made him fear for the survival of the republic and the lofty political concepts on which it was based.

Two days after he had treated his first case of yellow fever, he wrote to his wife, Julia, who was in Princeton, New Jersey, visiting her parents. He reported that he had lost three patients in two days and was treating another half dozen or so who appeared to be on the road to recovery. Days later, he wrote another letter, offering a grimmer vision of the situation. The disease, he wrote, "not only mocks in most instances the power of medicine, but it has spread through several parts of the city remote from the spot where it originated." The horrible scenes he witnessed, he wrote, reminded him of the stories he had read of the plague: "five other persons died in the neighborhood yesterday afternoon and four more last night at Kensington." Later, he recalled, "heaven alone bore witness to the anguish of my soul in this awful situation."[1]

Rush's anguish over the disease was confounded by hostility from most of the city's eighty physicians who openly ridiculed Rush's diagnosis. They persisted in their position that the disease was one of several common fevers that struck the city every year during warm weather. It would pass, all in good time, they argued. Dr. William Currie, who believed that the disease had been brought to Philadelphia by immigrants from the Caribbean and was spread from person to person, was among those who opposed Rush. His clinical description of the disease and its various stages is chilling in its detail:

> The symptoms which characterized the first stage of the fever, were, in the greatest number of cases, after a chilly fit of some duration, a quick, tense pulse—hot skin—pain in the head, back and limbs—flushed countenance—inflamed eye—moist tongue—oppression and sense of soreness at the stomach, especially upon pressure—frequent sick qualms, and retchings to vomit, without discharging anything, except the contents last taken into the stomach—costiveness [constipation]. And when stools were procured, the first generally showed a defect of bile, or an obstruction to its entrance into the intestines. But brisk purges generally altered this appearance [causing the stools to become darker].

These symptoms generally continued with more or less violence from one to three, four, or even five days; and then gradually abating, left the patient free from every complaint, except general debility. On the febrile symptoms suddenly subsiding, they were immediately succeeded by a yellow tinge in the opaque cornea, or whites of the eyes—and increased oppression at the praecordia—a constant puking of everything taken into the stomach, with much straining, accompanied by a hoarse hollow noise. . . .

The febrile symptoms, however, as has been already observed, either gave way on the third, fourth, or fifth days, and then the patient recovered; or they were soon after succeeded by a different, but much more dangerous train of symptoms, by debility, low pulse, cold skin (which assumed a tawny color, mixed with purple), black vomiting, hemorrhages, hiccups, anxiety, restlessness, coma. Many, who survived the eighth day, though apparently out of danger, died suddenly in consequence of a hemorrhage.[2]

It is helpful to remember that medicine, as practiced in the late 1700s, was not so much a science as it was an art, and as such it was influenced by human emotions that have influenced art since time began. Since physicians knew nothing about bacteria or viruses, they looked for linkages to society as a whole. Thus, a sick body was linked to a sick economy or sick government, the health of each intertwined with invisible forces that controlled their lives. Rush was obsessed with the symbolism that he saw overlapping in the two great passions of his life—medicine and politics.

Thirteen years after the Philadelphia epidemic, Rush wrote a revealing letter to John Adams in which he suggested that his remedies for yellow fever—purging and bloodletting—do "wonders" with some political leaders: "Ten and ten [as our doses of calomel and jalap were called in 1793] would be a substitute for a fistula in the bowels of Bonaparte. Bleeding would probably lessen the rage for altering the Constitution of Pennsylvania in the leaders of the party who are not contending for that measure. Tonics might be useful to those persons who behold with timidity the insults and spoliations that are offered to our commerce. The cold bath might cure the peevish irritability of some of the members of our Congress, and blisters and mustard plasters rouse the apathy of others. In short, there is a great field opened for new means of curing moral and political maladies."[3]

In late August, the College of Physicians of Philadelphia met to discuss options for the city's medical community. The membership voted to create a special commission—Rush was one of four physicians named—to write a report, due the following day, on the best means to treat and prevent the spread of yellow fever.

After the meeting, Rush hurried home in the rain to write the report, a task that took him most of the night. He and the other committee members returned the next day and read the report, which was adopted unanimously by the membership. Copies were sent to elected officials and to newspapers. The report consisted of nine measures of prevention and protection:

- Avoid every infected person as much as possible.
- Avoid fatigue of body and mind. Don't stand or sit in a draft, in the sun, or in the evening air.
- Dress according to the weather. Avoid intemperance. Drink sparingly of wine, beer, or cider.
- When visiting the sick, use vinegar or camphor on your handkerchief; carry it in smelling bottles; use it frequently.
- Somehow mark every house with sickness in it, on the door or window.
- Place your patients in the center of your biggest, airiest room in beds without curtains. Change their clothes and bed linen often. Remove all offensive matter as quickly as possible.
- Clean the streets, and keep them clean.
- Stop building fires in your houses or on the streets. They

have no useful effect. But burn gunpowder. It clears the air. And use vinegar and camphor generally.

- Most important of all, let a large and airy hospital be provided near the city to receive poor people stricken with the disease who cannot otherwise be cared for.[4]

Physicians were not the only Philadelphians who engaged in the public debate about yellow fever. Mayor Matthew Clarkson placed a notice in the newspapers warning that there was "great reason to apprehend that a dangerous infectious disorder" was afoot in the city. Fearing that the stench of rotting animals could be contributing to the epidemic, he ordered city workers to clean the streets of dead animals and decaying garbage. Pennsylvania governor Thomas Mifflin, who was scheduled to address an upcoming meeting of the state legislature, asked health officers to prepare a report to inform lawmakers and citizens of the progress of the disease.

Meanwhile, as the city's physicians and political leaders debated the causes of the disease, the death rate escalated day by day so that, by the end of August, nearly three hundred deaths could be attributed to the epidemic. When word of the epidemic reached other communities, Philadelphia refugees were sometimes greeted with hostility. Postmasters in surrounding states dipped all mail originating in Philadelphia in vinegar, handling each and every envelope with a pair of tongs. Newspapers and pamphlets from the city often were soaked in vinegar and then dried over an open fire before they were deemed safe to read.

*   *   *

Bodies littered the streets, festering in the hot sun and surrounded by dense clouds of flies. The air was so thick with illness that it sometimes was difficult to breathe. On one occasion, passersby spotted a sailor stretched out in the street and called for the carter, afraid to get too close to the corpse. As the sailor was being dragged away for burial, he roused from his drunken stupor and protested his removal with howls that sent a shiver throughout the entire neighborhood. A man and his wife were found dead in their bed, a baby lying between them still sucking at its dead mother's breast. A woman ordered a coffin for her dead husband, but then refused it because she felt it was too cheap. Instead, she purchased a more expensive model, only to die herself the following week and be buried in the cheap coffin she had rejected. A man returned home to find his wife unconscious and, believing she was dead, fled to avoid contamination. The next morning, he returned with a coffin only to find her recovered from the illness. A few days later, he died and was buried in the coffin he selected for his wife.[5] And so the madness went, day after day, week after week, as the emotional anguish associated with suffering and death competed with yellow fever itself as a conduit for terror.

As September began, Dr. Benjamin Rush wrote to a physician in Trenton, New Jersey, that he felt certain that the worst was over. He attributed his success with the disease to the calomel purgative that he gave patients to empty their bowels. Later that day, he dashed off a note to the Philadelphia College of Physicians in which he expressed confidence that he had found the long-awaited cure for yellow fever. So confident was he of the drug's effectiveness that he began telling desperately ill patients that they "only" had yellow fever, nothing to worry about.

By mid-September, Rush's optimism was dashed by reports that the city's death toll had risen to more than forty persons per day—that should not have come as a shock since he alone was treating more than one hundred patients each day—and by the harsh realization that he himself had come down with the disease. "My body became highly impregnated with the contagion," he wrote. "My eyes were yellow, and sometimes a yellowness was perceptible in my face." When he was able to sleep, he often awoke to find his bedding soaked with his own sweat. "These sweats were so offensive as to oblige me to draw the bedclothes close to my neck, to defend myself from their smell."[6]

Rush instructed his assistants to administer his purgative and bloodletting "cure" to him, and within a week he was again seeing patients in his home. So many people arrived at his home that he was forced to draft his five assistants into service as nurses, with each man seeing more than thirty patients a day. The traffic was so heavy that they quickly ran out of vessels to hold the blood they drew from the patients, making it necessary for them to perform the bloodletting outside, where the blood could flow through the paving stones of the road.

Despite his illness, Rush soon resumed his rounds, struggling through exhaustion and fever to treat his patients. When word of his illness spread through the community, there was panic among the uninfected. Without Rush to treat them, what would become of them if they fell ill? In fact, most of the other physicians already had fled the city and sought refuge in the countryside.

The epidemic presented a dilemma to President Washington. One day his wife, Martha, went shopping with Polly Lear, his personal assistant's wife, after which she came down with a fever. A few weeks later, Martha wrote to a friend, "We have had a melancholy time hear [sic] for about a fortnight past Mrs. Lear was taken with a fever—the doctor was called in but to no purpose her illness increased until the eighth day she was taken from us—she never lost her senses till just before she expired—Mr. Lear bares [sic] his loss like a philosopher—she is generally lamented by all that knew her." The president was one of the pallbearers at her funeral.[7]

Washington insisted that Martha take the children and go to Mount Vernon, but she refused to leave Philadelphia without him. He felt that it was unseemly for the president to leave the city while other men and women remained. It was a matter of duty, he argued. Very well, she responded, if duty was the most important thing in the world, then she and the children would remain in the city to do their "duty." He made arrangements for Martha and the children to leave the city with an escort, but she stood firm in her decision not to leave without him. Finally, weary of arguing with her about it, he relented and agreed to leave.

For most Philadelphians, the seriousness of the situation did not fully sink in until a three-line newspaper item announced that Philadelphia's most prominent citizen, President George Washington, had left the city to return to his home in Mount Vernon. Wrote Washington to a friend: "It was my wish to have continued here longer, but as Mrs. Washington was unwilling to leave me surrounded by the malignant fever which prevailed. I could not think of hazarding her and the children any longer by my continuance in the city the house in which we lived being, in a manner, blockaded by the disorder and was becoming every day more and more fatal."

Washington felt bad about abandoning the city in a time of peril, but the decision was made somewhat easier by the fact that the government was collapsing all around him. Secretary of the Treasury Alexander Hamilton, the president's main supporter, had come down with the fever, as had his wife. Washington's personal secretary, Tobias Lear, had left the city. The post office was shut down, and the Treasury Department was so depleted of staff that it was on the verge of collapse, held together by the stubborn work ethic of a single clerk who refused to abandon his post, even though his own daughter had died of the disease.

Before leaving Philadelphia, Washington met with Secretary of State Thomas Jefferson, who informed him that he, too, was preparing to leave, and he met with Secretary of War Henry Knox, whom he put in charge of the government. He instructed Knox to send a weekly report on the progress of the disease, and he recommended that the entire war department office be moved to a location away from the city. Concluded Washington: "I sincerely wish, and pray, that you and yours, may escape untouched and, when we meet again, that it may be under circumstances more pleasing than the present."

Throughout it all, African American immigrants from the West Indies continued to pour into the city. At the time of the first census in 1790, Philadelphia had the largest number of free African Americans in the United States, composing nearly five percent of the city's total population. It was considered a hospitable place for men and women of color, at least by the rigid standards of the day.

When Rush learned that many of the African American immigrants seemed to have a natural immunity to yellow fever, he showed them how to perform the bloodletting procedure and sent them out into the community to drain blood from patients. Age was no barrier to learning the skill. Rush's eleven-year-old servant boy was also taught how to draw blood from the sick and dying.

To some, Rush seemed like a savior—and they flocked to his home office by the hundreds, begging for his assistance. However, to others he was deemed a madman and uncharitably dubbed the "Prince of Bleeders." The newspapers were filled with criticism and praise for the doctor, so much so that he became as much a topic of debate as the disease itself. When an irate citizen told a newspaper that Rush had made "one of those great discoveries which have contributed to the depopulation of the earth," the doctor responded that the only people dying in Philadelphia were those too poor to afford medical care and those in the upper classes who received their care from his detractors. Annoyed by the criticisms, Rush wrote his wife and complained that, in addition to struggling with yellow fever, he was forced to contend with the "prejudices, fears, and falsehoods of several of my brethren, all of which retard the progress of truth and daily cost our city many lives."[8]

Also filling the newspapers were political debates about the cause of the epidemic. Republicans maintained that the disease was caused by local factors, while Federalists blamed the ships that arrived from foreign ports, and Federalists used the disease as an excuse to block trade with the French, especially as it applied to goods imported from French-controlled islands. Republicans interpreted the Federalist position as an attack against their right to trade with the West Indies.

Complicating the political argument was Dr. Currie's assertion that the disease had originated aboard a French ship that had arrived in Philadelphia in July. Federalists used Currie's opinion as proof that Republicans were engaged in a sinister cover-up to protect their financial links to the French. Furthermore, they charged that Republicans concocted their theory of a local cause of the disease as part of a plot to discredit the city and relocate the capital to a more rural setting. Republicans denied that allegation and said that they wanted to save cities through sanitary reform, not destroy them. A mob mentality developed on the street as rumors persisted that the city's wells had been contaminated prior to a French invasion. Conspiracy theories abounded. Citizens were warned not to trust French doctors for fear they were part of a sinister plot to seize control of the city.

Not immune to the politics of the day, Benjamin Rush identified the Federalists' criticisms of his cures with the French Revolution, comparing his situation to that of the French Republic, "surrounded and invaded by new as well as old enemies, without any other allies." He maintained that the cure for yellow fever would be determined by the will of the majority and not by political elitists.

Running parallel to the politics of the epidemic was a religious viewpoint that yellow fever had been inflicted by God upon the city as retribution for its collective sins. The pious pointed to a series of "sins" that the city had committed, including the construction of a new performance theater that detractors dubbed the "Synagogue for Satan." They saw the building, which contained ornaments made of pure gold and fluted marble columns, as a symbol of evil. They said it resembled a palace more than it did a theater, and they compared it to a bordello. Since the theater's major backers were Federalists, Republicans used the theater to rally the pious to their side. Not until the Federalists changed their evils ways, argued the Republicans, would the city's good health be restored by God.

A pious man himself, Rush suggested that God had singled him out to combat the epidemic. His religious history had been erratic—he went from Episcopalian to Presbyterian, then to Universalist, and back again to Episcopalian—but he began each day with a devotional, prayed often, and encouraged others to pray, and he read from the Bible as time permitted, but always on a daily basis. To his wife, he wrote, "It is meat and drink to me to do my Master's will. He loved human life, and among other errands into our world, he came not to destroy men's lives but to save them." If he was on a mission from God, Rush reflected, how could he possibly fail?

*   *   *

In an effort to prove themselves to the white residents, the city's nearly three thousand blacks, under the impression that they were immune to the disease because of their African ancestry, decided to remain behind and care for the sick and dying. They assisted Dr. Benjamin Rush, at his request, performing hundreds of bloodletting procedures and keeping copious notes on all their cases—and they bravely manned the carts that traveled the city to pick up the corpses.

White Philadelphians were glad to see them when loved ones were ill, or when there had been a death in the family, for no whites could be persuaded to touch the graying and bloated corpses, but once the dirty work was done, they averted their eyes and fled from any blacks they saw on the street, fearful that they might be contaminated. A printer named Mathew Carey published a book titled *A Short Account of the Malignant Fever, Lately Prevalent in Philadelphia*, in which he accused the blacks who worked as nurses, gravediggers, and undertakes of thievery and assorted other crimes.

Eventually, complaints reached Mayor Clarkson that the blacks were charging exorbitant rates for their work, and he met with black leaders to discuss the matter. He was told that blacks did not have fixed rates for their work and accepted what they were given, often working for no payment at all. As it turned out, the stories of high rates were caused by a handful of whites who offered the blacks large sums to care for their sick and to bury their dead. Two of the black leaders who met with the mayor, Absalom Jones and Richard Allen, later wrote a book about black experiences during the epidemic titled *A Narrative of the Proceedings of the Black People, during the Late Awful Calamity in Philadelphia, in the Year 1793: and a Refutation of Some Censures, Thrown upon Them in Some Late Publications*. The book reported instances in which blacks witnessed a white nurse stealing buckles and other valuables from a couple who had died on the same night, and it told about an elderly lady's white nurse who had died, lying drunk, with the patient's rings on her fingers and in her pockets. On the other hand, the book reported instances in which black workers went from one house to another, taking only what was offered. A young black woman refused to take money because she felt that God would punish her for it and afflict her with the disease. An elderly black woman, when asked her price for caring for a loved one, answered, "a dinner, master, on a cold winter's day."[9]

Of course, the only blacks who had immunity to yellow fever were those who had traveled to America from infected areas in Africa or the Caribbean where they would have been exposed to the disease at a young age and escaped with no symptoms or minor symptoms that allowed their bodies to produce antibodies. Once African Americans began dying of the disease, Rush took note: "If the disorder would continue to spread among them, then will the measure of our suffering be full."

The debate over whether African Americans were unfairly profiting from the misery of whites must be viewed within the context of the times. As an institution, slavery was thriving— indeed, George Washington had staffed the Executive Mansion with slaves he brought from his Virginia plantation. Without ever mentioning slavery, the Constitution protected the rights of slave owners with Section 3 of Article IV, which read: "No person held to Service or Labour in one State, escaping into another, shall, in Consequence of any Law or Regulation therein, be discharged from such Service or Labour, but shall be delivered up on Claim of the Party to whom such Service or Labour may be due." Only months before the yellow fever epidemic hit, Washington signed into law the Fugitive Slave Act, which provided, in a more detailed way, the manner in which escaped slaves could be reclaimed by their masters. In essence, the law stated that a slave owner could legally seize a runaway and take him before a judge in the jurisdiction where he was captured. After proof of owner-ship was provided, the judge was required to issue an order per-mitting the slave's return. The law made slaves fair game for bounty hunters who tracked down fugitives for a fee.

Philadelphia's black population was composed of slaves, free men and women, and newly arrived immigrants from Africa and the West Indies, some of whom were free and some of whom were slaves. Opinions about slavery were as divisive in the city as they were elsewhere in the country. Benjamin Franklin, who had signed the Declaration of Independence, and then had served as a delegate to the constitutional convention, was the outspoken president of the Pennsylvania Society for Promoting the Abolition of Slavery. He died three years before the arrival of the 1793 epi-demic, but his opinions about the institution of slavery still car-ried weight in the city.

Pro-slavery Philadelphians, especially those who did not own slaves, reacted with bitterness to the sight of African Americans being paid to nurse sick whites and to cart away dead bodies. Shouldn't that work be done, they argued, by slaves? Antislavery Philadelphians pointed out that people who owned slaves would never allow their valuable investments to be exposed to yellow fever, unless, of course, their help was required to nurse family members back to health. They argued that the city's free blacks were performing a valuable service, and so what if they made a dollar or two in the process—wasn't that free enterprise at work? Philadelphians, already stressed by the ravages of yellow fever, allowed racism and politics to further contaminate the atmosphere, giving free rein to paranoia as the sole arbiter of discourse in the city.

*   *   *

Working out of his office at Mount Vernon, President George Washington spent most days in frustration, isolated from the levers of power. His biggest problem was that he had none of the files he needed to carry on with the business of government. Although he had left Secretary of War Henry Knox in charge of the government in his absence, Knox himself fled the city only days after Washington's departure and traveled to Manhattan, where he was turned away because of his exposure to yellow fever. He ended up in Elizabethtown, New Jersey, where town officials put him under quarantine for two weeks. Knox wrote to him every week, as promised, but not from Philadelphia.

Washington felt paralyzed. Typical of the problems that arose was an incident involving the British-owned ship *Roehampton*, which was seized by the French and brought into Baltimore Harbor. The British demanded that Washington release the ship to them, and the French demanded that he give the ship to them. Embarrassed by his lack of legal information, Washington told the Maryland governor, Thomas Lee, that he was unable to make an immediate decision. "I brought no public papers of any sort (not even the rules which have been established in these cases), along with me," he wrote to Lee. "Consequently, [I] am not prepared at this place to decide points which may require a reference to papers not within my reach."[10]

Complicating everything else was the fact that he needed to call Congress into session, but there were legal questions about whether he could do that in a location outside of Philadelphia. He wrote all his cabinet officers to ask their opinions, but there was no consensus about what he should do. Alexander Hamilton was among those arguing that the president had the power to assemble the government in any location he chose. To resolve the matter, Washington turned to the nation's top law officer, Attorney General Edmund Randolph, who advised the president that he did not have the power to relocate Congress. For him to do so, he wrote, would clearly be unconstitutional.

Unable to make a decision, Washington remained at Mount Vernon, where he paced and awaited each day's mail delivery, optimistic that events soon would turn his way. It was the biggest lesson he had learned to date: Leading an army required courage and daring, the willingness to make decisions and then to follow through with them, while leading a nation required compromise and careful decisions based, to some extent, on the quality of paperwork that he had at his disposal. Without paper, there could be no government—and, for the moment at least, he was a pauper in that regard.

Meanwhile, in Philadelphia, the epidemic showed promise of ending with the first frost. In October, Washington received a letter from Postmaster General Timothy Pickering that cold weather had produced a cleansing effect in the city. At mid-month, deaths were averaging 120 per day, but within a week that number had been cut in half. Pickering wrote that Benjamin Rush had assured him that the epidemic would be over by December 2, the date that Congress was scheduled to convene.

On October 28, Washington boarded a coach, along with Tobias Lear and a valet, and began the five-day trip to Philadelphia. Later, they were joined in Baltimore by Thomas Jefferson, who shared a private coach with them to a small town just outside Philadelphia. Washington had made prior arrangements to stay in a private residence, which meant that Jefferson had to go from inn to inn until he could find a vacancy—and, even then, all he could find was a small, unfurnished room without a bed, a table, or a chair in the King of Prussia tavern. Jefferson was miserable and complained at every opportunity.

Gradually, the news reports out of Philadelphia provided optimism that the city soon would return to normal. As his yellow fever cases trickled down to a few, Benjamin Rush, who by then spent most of his time reading and making notes about his cases, found himself in a reflective mood. "Sometimes seated in your easy chair by the fire," he wrote to Julia, "I lose myself in looking back upon the ocean which I have passed, and now and then find myself surprised by a tear in reflecting upon the friends I have lost, and the scenes of distress that I have witnessed and which I was unable to relieve."[11]

Washington came under increased pressure to convene Congress at a location outside of Philadelphia, but he was not convinced that he should do so. On November 10, Washington rose early and asked for his horse. Without telling anyone where he was going, he rode alone into Philadelphia to see for himself if the city was returning to normal. He was pleased by what he saw: a city that was awakening, as if from a long sleep, with people filling the streets, going about the business of living. When he returned and told his staff about his trip, they were horrified that he would venture out alone without protection, but they were pleased that he had decided not to relocate Congress.

On November 14, Pennsylvania governor Thomas Mifflin issued a proclamation establishing December 12 as a day of "general humiliation, thanksgiving and prayer." Published in newspapers across the state, it proclaimed: "Whereas it hath pleased Almighty God to put an end to the grievous Calamity, that recently afflicted the City of Philadelphia, and it is the Duty of all . . . to employ the earliest moments of returning Health, in devout expressions of penitence, humiliation and gratitude."

Not long after Washington returned to Philadelphia, he sent for Martha and the children, convinced that cooler weather had made the city safe to inhabit. However, their homecoming was not without sorrow, for they found a traumatized city in which many of their old friends were dead. Like most Philadelphians, they yearned for everything to return to normal but found that it was a slow process, complicated by the emotional healing that was necessary in the wake of so much death and destruction.

In January 1794, about six weeks after her return, Martha wrote to a friend: "They have suffered so much that it can not be got over soon by those that was [sic] in the city—almost every family has lost some of their friends—and black seems to be the general dress of the city—the [theater] players are not allowed to come here nor has there been any assembly." The following month, she wrote that the river was frozen and the air was very cold: "A great number of people in this town is [sic] very much at a loss how to spend their time agreeably. The gay are always fond of some new scenes let it be what it may—I dare say a very little time will ware [sic] of the gloom if gay amusements are permitted here."[12]

By the time yellow fever finally ran its course, it had claimed the lives of more than four thousand Philadelphians, giving the city the distinction of hosting the largest yellow fever epidemic in the nation's history. To put it in a modern-day perspective, the death toll would be the equivalent of New York City losing 1.1 million citizens in the infamous September 11, 2001, terrorist attack. The survivors were indelibly marked for life. Dr. Benjamin Rush, who did as much as any individual to combat the epidemic, was embittered and discouraged by the experience. He was especially disappointed with the College of Physicians, which had not

supported him in his conclusions about yellow fever and had promoted a "conspiracy" against him. Though he had helped found
the organization, he submitted his resignation, enclosing a book
by an innovative British physician whose conclusions about the
disease had mirrored his own.

Even before the epidemic made Philadelphia into a ghost
town, George Washington had argued that a city that size was not
a proper location for the seat of government. He felt that the
nation's capital should be located in a rural area, far away from
the diseases and social problems that afflicted cities. For the site
of the new capital, he chose a parcel of land offered by Maryland
state officials. Located on the Potomac River on land that had
been seized from the Conoy Indians, it was bordered by Maryland
and Virginia. The nearest city was Baltimore, thirty-eight miles to
the southeast.

In the wake of the 1793 epidemic, Washington was given a
free hand by Congress to create the District of Columbia, a decision that was viewed with increasing satisfaction as yellow fever
returned to Philadelphia for lesser epidemics in 1794, 1796, 1797,
1798—right up until 1800, when the north section of the capitol
was completed, providing lawmakers with a permanent summer
refuge from the ravages of urban yellow fever.

CHAPTER TWO

new orleans

gateway to death

In 1718, four years after the French set up a trading post in Natchez, Mississippi, Jean Baptiste Le Moyne, Sieur de Bienville, followed the river south to establish a settlement on Indian camping grounds. The settlement, built on the east bank of the Mississippi River, ninety miles from the river's mouth but more than one hundred miles from the Gulf of Mexico, was named Nouvelle Orleans (New Orleans) after the Duke of Orleans. It was a swampy patch of land, filled with alligators, poisonous snakes, and buzzing mosquitoes. The water table was so high that it was impossible to build basements or dig graves, making it necessary for burials—and there were plenty in those days—to take place above ground in stone vaults.

Within four years, New Orleans became the capital of the expansive French province of Louisiana. French explorers used New Orleans as a base of operations until 1762, when the Louisiana Territory was given to Spain. The first recorded yellow fever epidemic in New Orleans occurred in 1796, just three years after the Philadelphia nightmare, but the disease kept a low profile until the turn of the century, by which time the French had forced war-weakened Spain to cede the territory back to France.

When that happened, President Thomas Jefferson, who was opposed to French expansion in North America, offered to buy

Florida from Spain, keeping his efforts a secret from Congress. When it became apparent that the land transfer would take place, he wrote to his envoy in Paris: "There is on the globe one single spot the possessor of which is our natural and habitual enemy. It is New Orleans. France placing herself in that door assumes to us the attitude of defiance. . . . [I find] it impossible that France and the U.S. can continue long friends when they meet in so irritable a position."[1]

To avert a war with France, Jefferson asked the American envoy in Paris to broker a deal. His preference was to purchase New Orleans, but, if that failed, the envoy was instructed to work out a treaty that would allow America continued use of the Mississippi River. To Jefferson's surprise, France offered to sell the entire Louisiana Territory, all 875,000 acres, to the United States for $15 million. The envoy accepted the offer, and the treaty setting forth the land transfer was dated April 30, 1803.

To most of the world, the Louisiana Territory was little more than an inhospitable swamp at its southernmost tip, a vast wilderness that radiated northward to Canada and westward to the Rocky Mountains into heavily forested Indian lands that were of no apparent value to anyone in the Western world, but, to Jefferson, the Louisiana Territory was critical to America's expansion of what he called its "empire of liberty."

By 1803 New Orleans was an important port, with ships arriving from all over the world, many of them bringing slaves from Africa, or from Georgia and Virginia, to be sold and shipped up river to Natchez and Memphis. At one time, the city boasted more than two dozen slave-auction houses. The slaves not sent to work the plantations were used as domestics and ultimately played a major role in the development of the city's social and music heritage. New Orleans soon possessed one of the largest populations of people of color in the South, largely because of the sexual experimentation that took place among whites, black slaves, and Indians. In time, the people of mixed color began calling themselves Creoles to set themselves apart from the boat-loads of immigrants that arrived on a regular basis from Ireland. Creoles went into journeyman professions such as cigar-making and bricklaying, building a solid middle class that became the foundation of French Quarter society. They spent their money freely, put a special emphasis on dressing well, and sometimes sent their children to France to be educated in the best schools.

Despite the city's change in ownership, the French influence remained strong, especially in cuisine, architecture, and enter-tainment. Today the French Quarter runs from Canal Street to Esplanade, covering an area of approximately one hundred thirty square blocks, a showplace of architecture that dates almost back to the beginning, when French builders strived to duplicate the triumphs of Paris with buildings that offered courtyards that, although magnificent in design and ambiance, provided fertile environments for mosquito procreation.

In January 1819, New Orleans was host to a most distin-guished visitor—architect Benjamin Henry Latrobe, father of the Greek Revival style in America and designer of the US capitol in Washington. Born in England, he worked in Germany and France before coming to America, gaining experience that provided him with a worldly view of American society. He was interested in New Orleans because of its reputation as a world-class port and the French architecture that characterized the heralded down-town French Quarter. Despite his expectations, what impressed Latrobe the most was not the city's architecture but rather its cacophony of exotic sounds. As far as his eye could see, there were shopkeepers out on the street loudly advertising their wares, everything from bananas to rare books. Later, he wrote that some of the shopkeepers had stalls and tables, but most had their wares laid out on the ground: "The articles to be sold were not more var-ious than the Sellers. White men and women, and of all hues of brown, and of all Classes of faces, from round Yankees, to grisly and lean Spaniards, black Negroes and negresses, filthy Indians half naked, Mulattoes, curly and straight-haired and frizzled, the women dressed in the most flaring yellow and scarlet gowns the men capped and hated. . . . I cannot suppose that my eye took in less than five hundred sellers and buyers, all of whom appeared to strain their voices, to exceed each other in loudness."

Convinced that New Orleans was unique among cities, Latrobe left with an exuberant impression of the people and the city's potential for growth. Visitors like Latrobe who then returned home to write glowingly about their adventures were responsible for the arrival of boatloads of immigrants from Europe, most of whom were hungry for exotic new lives.

With the growth of the city's port and the arrival of immigrants from the Caribbean, yellow fever returned to New Orleans, slowly at first—with minor appearances in 1812, 1817, and 1818 that claimed fewer than three hundred lives. It was not until 1819 that the disease again escalated to major status, with an epidemic that killed more than two thousand, a sizable portion of the city's twenty-six thousand citizens. Little note was taken of the epidemic in the rest of the country, primarily because New Orleans was still viewed as a frontier outpost where bad things were expected to happen to good people on a regular basis.

Beginning in 1822, yellow fever returned to New Orleans every year for twenty-five years, sometimes killing as few as five persons, as in 1826, and other times killing several hundred (239 in 1823, 215 in 1829, 210 in 1833, 412 in 1837, and 594 in 1841). Not until 1847 did another major epidemic appear, claiming 2,306 lives.

Health officials found it a troublesome disease, not just because of its high mortality rate, but because the medical community was unable to agree on the causes and treatment of the disease, and public perception was often at odds with any positions taken by the medical establishment. Dr. Benjamin Rush of Philadelphia was considered the leading authority, with recent validation of Rush's position offered by French physician

Nicholas Cherbin, who argued that yellow fever was not contagious and could not be diminished with quarantines. As proof, Rush and Cherbin offered the observation that, when people fled an epidemic, they did not take the disease with them to other towns and communities. In Rush's and Cherbin's minds, the disease was clearly rooted in time and place.

Public opinion was clearly on the side of quarantines. Regardless of what physicians said, ordinary citizens shunned people with the disease—indeed, they were afraid to touch a yellow fever victim, living or dead—and supported the imposition of quarantines, sometimes to the point of making it a political issue. That attitude was one reason the city council voted in 1826 to prohibit funeral services from being held at the city's showcase church, St. Louis Cathedral. Instead, a new funeral chapel was built near the St. Louis Cemetery at a cost of fourteen thousand dollars, far enough away from the cathedral to give church members peace of mind.

Of course, church funerals were only for the most fortunate. The ordeal was a nightmare for ministers who found themselves in daily contact with the afflicted. Wrote Presbyterian minister Theodore Clapp: "Often I have met and shook hands with some blooming, handsome young man today, and in a few hours afterward, I have been called to see him with profuse hemorrhages from the mouth, nose, ears, eyes, and even toes; the eyes prominent, glistening, yellow and staring; the face discolored with orange color and dusky red."[2] Typically, well-to-do yellow fever victims were buried above ground in vaults, but the less-well-off were dumped into shallow ditches near where they died, without benefit of religious rites. The idea was to get infected corpses underground as quickly as possible, but not so deep into the ground that the ditch would fill with water. No doubt, many of the "corpses" that were rushed to the ditch were still alive and died from suffocation instead of infection, but those were the risks that people took when they isolated themselves from family and friends in their time of sickness.

As the nineteenth century approached the halfway point, yellow fever epidemics mysteriously disappeared in the northern states while increasing in frequency in the South, leading to public prejudice in the North that the South was disease-ridden and backward, incapable of sustaining a thriving economy. Yellow fever was called the "Stranger's Disease," meaning that travelers to the South were more likely to get infected than the indigenous population. There was some truth to that since children who were exposed to the disease often came down with minor infections that allowed them to build an immunity that protected them in adulthood. But no one understood that aspect of the disease at the time, and the "Stranger's Disease" soon assumed all the trappings of social stigma. It was a burden that the South carried for another century at least.

*   *   *

In 1810, New Orleans had a population of ten thousand. By 1850, the city's population had soared to 116,375, spurred by revolutions in Europe that sent French and German immigrants to the city, and by the Irish potato famine, which sent tens of thousands of Irish laborers to the city, making New Orleans America's third-largest city, behind New York and Baltimore. The main reasons for the city's population explosion were the cotton and slave trades, which made its port the fourth busiest in the world. By 1850, cotton was a $100-million-a-year industry, representing an annual shipment of more than two million bales, with most of the cotton shipped to Liverpool and other European ports.

Along with the city's population surge came a need for more construction. New buildings had to be erected, and the swamps had to be drained and encircled by levees to protect the city from the Mississippi River, which flows at a higher level than most of the land in New Orleans. Most of that work was done by Irish laborers, many of whom arrived with typhus and other diseases.

Corresponding with the workers' arrival were the largest typhus outbreaks in Louisiana history. As a result, city hospitals filled with typhus patients at a rate of about eighteen thousand a year, almost all of them immigrants.

During the construction boom, there were more than ten thousand slaves residing in the city, but they were considered much too valuable to squander on construction work. Male slaves sold for about $2,000 at that time, about $20,000 in today's dollars, and female slaves fetched, on average, about $1,800. They were trained for skilled professions, such as blacksmithing, or used as household servants in what was essentially a protective environment. Few New Orleans residents could afford to own more than a few slaves, which meant that, when a family bought a slave, it represented a significant investment. Why subject a valuable slave to dangerous labor, slave owners reasoned, when newly arrived Irishmen and Germans were happy to do the work for pennies a day?

Following the 1847 yellow fever epidemic, the disease seemed to gradually recede, killing only 808 people in 1848, 769 in 1849, 107 in 1850, and a mere seventeen in 1851. A wave of relief swept through the city in 1851, and longtime New Orleans residents talked openly, if cautiously, about the possibility that the city had finally outgrown such a primitive disease. New Orleans competed with New York as the most cosmopolitan and economically vibrant city in the country, and city leaders were eager to put its swampy, frontier town image behind them.

Early in 1853, with the publication of the city directory, the editor wrote an editorial that praised Mayor A. D. Crossman for his leadership: "Five consecutive summers have now elapsed, since the scourge. . . . Yellow Fever in New Orleans is now considered by the faculty an 'obsolete idea.'"[3]

The preceding winter had been unusually successful, with more than $130 million in produce, mostly cotton, making its way down the river to New Orleans for distribution worldwide.

Because the weather had been favorable for shipping, New Orleans exporters wrapped up their business earlier than usual and set out for their summer residences in May in an effort to escape the worst of the summer heat in the city. Caught up in the excitement of the day, the *Daily Picayune* editorialized that "Nature has placed no limits to her [New Orleans'] greatness, she must become one of the largest cities in the world, perhaps one day the greatest commercial emporium on the face of the earth."

As May drew to a close, there were signs of trouble ahead, but no one wanted to give them serious attention, for to do so would be to deny the city's glorious future on the world stage. On May 27, a newly arrived Irish worker was admitted to Charity Hospital suffering from jaundice and black vomit. He died within hours. By chance, Dr. Erasmus Darwin Fenner, an authority on yellow fever, was the attending physician. He feared that his patient had died of yellow fever, but since the man's symptoms were not unlike those of other ailments, such as hepatitis and liver cancer, he was slow to make a diagnosis that would send the city into a panic. There was an understanding in the medical community that, before the dreaded "yellow fever" phrase could be uttered by a physician, it behooved him to identify several instances of the infection and to receive the support of several colleagues. Otherwise, any mention of the disease would be greeted by instant hostility from the city's newspapers and political establishment, thus making the management of an epidemic extremely difficult.

Before saying anything, Fenner looked for other suspicious cases, finding several that he thought could be attributed to yellow fever. Doing the work of an investigative reporter, Fenner checked the backgrounds of each patient, tracing the first cases to the ship *Augusta*, which had arrived in New Orleans from Bremen on May 17 with 230 European immigrants. He found nothing unusual about the ship's voyage to New Orleans, except two children who died of diarrhea. Fennel then turned his attention to a second ship, the *Camboden Castle*. After interviewing the captain, he learned that the ship's previous captain and several crew members died of yellow fever while docked in Kingston, Jamaica. However, no problems were reported on the ship during its voyage to New Orleans.

Fenner sought out the person who treated the suspected yellow fever cases aboard the *Augusta*, a well-known physician named Dr. Moritz Schuppert. The first man Schuppert treated, a twenty-one-year-old sailor who complained of headache, a rapid pulse, nausea, and vomiting, was diagnosed as having gastroduodenitis. His skin and eyes turned yellow on the fifth day, but then he recovered a few days later. Two days later, a second sailor became ill. He reported similar symptoms and died a few days later while in a state of delirium. Within days, two additional sailors developed similar symptoms, with one recovering and the other dying on May 30. Dr. Schuppert completed a postmortem and discovered that the man was yellow and his stomach contained two ounces of black vomit. A fifth victim from the ship became ill and died one week later.

Fenner consulted with his colleagues about the cases, but he found no agreement among them that yellow fever had caused the deaths. Meanwhile, a butcher who lived near the dock where the *Augusta* was moored came down with a similar disease that was marked by large quantities of black vomit. The butcher recovered, but Fenner was convinced that the man had been infected with yellow fever. When he went to his colleagues for confirmation, they were unable to agree on his diagnosis.

Within days, other suspicious cases began appearing in Charity Hospital. An Irish immigrant who had unloaded the ship docked next to the *Augusta* was admitted to the hospital on May 27, only to die the following morning. At the postmortem, attended by Fenner and several of his colleagues, there was full agreement that the man had died of yellow fever. Of course, Fenner's investigative effort tried to track the cause of yellow fever to its root, but that never happened. He was like most other physicians of that era in that he desperately wanted to acquire a better understanding of the disease and solve its mystery. Fenner authored a book about his experiences, *History of the Epidemic Yellow Fever at New Orleans, La., 1853*, which was published in 1854, but even after an exhaustive investigation, he still had no more of an idea about what caused yellow fever or how it was transmitted than when he began his inquiry.

Yellow fever marched with relentless determination through June, never claiming enough victims on a given day—no more than two dozen in a week—to justify a public declaration that an epidemic was in progress. Instead, it lurked in the shadows, sending a steady flow of patients to the hospital, where they either recovered within a week or so or died within days of arrival. Death from infectious disease, it must be remembered, was a common occurrence throughout America in the years before the arrival of antibiotics.

Despite continuing yellow fever cases, New Orleans slipped into a false sense of security. The times had changed since the last major epidemic in 1819, which was almost two generations removed from the city's current mood of invincibility. None of the native-born residents in their twenties and thirties had any memory of the terror associated with the 1819 epidemic, nor did any of the tens of thousands of new immigrants. As a result, New Orleans went through June in a state of public lethargy, seemingly without a care in the world.

The mood changed drastically in July. New Orleans went from twenty-five yellow fever deaths a week to more than five hundred deaths a week. The first inkling of trouble appeared in the city's newspapers, all of which had downplayed June's death figures out of a misplaced sense of civic responsibility. Why send the city into panic, publishers reasoned, if there is no evidence of an epidemic?

As the death toll escalated in July, the newspapers reconsidered their previous positions and determined that good journalism put a higher premium on the public's right to know than on the newspapers' devotion to civic boosterism, but they still slanted their news coverage in obvious ways. When the *Delta* reported high yellow fever death rates, it rationalized that most of the victims were Irish and German immigrants who had neglected medical care until it was too late, thus comforting native-born New Orleans residents, who felt they were not at risk because they were too knowledgeable about medical care to ever succumb to a lower-class disease such as yellow fever.

As the deaths continued, the *Delta* modified its position. After reporting on August 1 that the city had carried out 880 burials the previous week, 692 because of yellow fever, the newspaper admitted that it had been mistaken in its assessment that the medical community would be able to control the disease. After stating the obvious, the newspaper concluded, "We still have confidence that the worst day has arrived, and pray our readers to have patience for a few days, when we hope to be able to announce the gratifying fact of its rapid decline."

In an act of incredible political cowardice, the board of aldermen boldly resolved during the last week of July that yellow fever had not become epidemic in the city, immediately after which the board adjourned until October, allowing lawmakers to flee to a place of safety outside the city until the death toll subsided.

The only leadership that remained in the city came from physicians, ministers, and priests, who cared for the spiritual and physical needs of the public, often without regard to their own safety. Parson Theodore Clapp, a Protestant minister who served in New Orleans during the epidemic, later wrote:

When nearly all of the so-called better elements in the city had fled, physicians and clergymen held to their duty of ministering to the physical and spiritual wants of the people. Never, till I went to Louisiana, did I behold that living and most perfect exemplification of a Christian spirit exhibited in the conduct and benefactions of those denominated [Daughters] of Charity.

Look at them. They were, in many instances, born and bred in the lap of worldly ease and luxury. But in obedience to a sense of religious duty, they have relinquished the pleasures of time for the charms of a life consecrated to duty and to God.

There, calm and gentle as angels, they stay at their posts amid the most frightful epidemics, till death comes to take them to a better world. When I have seen them smoothing the pillow, and whispering the consolations of religion for some unfortunate fellow being, his last moments—dying among strangers, far from home, never again to behold the face of wife, child, relative or friend this side of the grave—I could hardly realize that they were beings of mortality. They seemed to me like ministering angels sent down from the realms of celestial glory.[4]

Nestled among the stories of heartwarming self-sacrifice and devotion to duty were stories of a darker nature, such as the old man, employed as a hospital nurse, who possessed a dark fascination with terminally ill patients. Each time he came across a patient writhing in agony, he chuckled at the sight of such pain, and, each time his patients reached the black-vomit stage, he grinned with what was described by observers as a "strange light." For him, there was no joy in life that did not involve the sight of his fellow man in pain. Even so, nurses willing to take care of yellow fever patients were in short supply, and the hospital apparently never gave any thought to replacing the crazed old man with a more compassionate worker.

With no effective political leadership in the city, residents broke up into what could be called benevolent vigilante groups—various organizations that conducted relief operations aimed at lessening the suffering of those afflicted with the disease. Some, such as the Howard Association, helped with drug and medical bills. Others, such as the Louisiana Grays, the Masonic Broad of Relief, and various fire stations, raised money for general purposes and gathered clothing and bed linens to aid stricken families.

To combat the epidemic, city officials fired six-pound cannons into the air (an attempt to "purify" the atmosphere) and burned barrels of tar at strategic locations around the city in an attempt to cleanse the air of disease. Wrote one diarist about the firing of cannon: "At sunset, when all were simultaneously fired, a pandemonium glare lighted up our city. Not a breath of air disturbed the dense smoke, which slowly ascended in curling columns until it reached the height of about five hundred feet. Here it seemed equipoised, festooning over our doomed city like a funeral pall, and there remaining until the shades of night disputed with it the reign of darkness."

One needed only to walk through the streets to understand the terror that accompanied the disease. "As we passed the cemeteries, we saw coffins piled up beside the gate and in the walks, and the laborers at work, digging trenches in preparation for the morrow's dead," wrote one resident. "A fog, which hung over the moss-covered oaks, prevented the egress of the dense and putrid exhalations. The atmosphere was nauseating to a degree that I have never noticed in a sick room."

In early August, the New Orleans Grand Jury issued a report that dealt with a number of pressing community matters, including yellow fever. Unable to determine a cause of the epidemic, the grand jury concluded that the city's poor sanitation habits were at fault for the spread of the disease. Especially troublesome, said the report, were the piles of dead animals, garbage, and filth that lined the streets. In conclusion, the grand jury noted: "The entire health or sanitary system is radically wrong."[5]

In August one could not walk very far along city streets without encountering a corpse, a funeral procession, or a building that echoed with moans and wails or without being overcome by the stench of death. One newspaper reporter wrote of a young girl, clad in an old mourning dress, walking in the hot sun behind a cart driven by a young boy, about ten or twelve, who shouted at his tired horse to keep him moving through the heat. The girl and little boy were all that was left of a family that had numbered half a dozen members. On that day, they were transporting their father to the cemetery, a two-mile walk that seemed certain to push them to exhaustion.

Many yellow fever victims were delayed in their journey to the grave. By midmonth, more than two hundred persons a day were dying of yellow fever. Grave diggers had so much work that they simply could not keep up with demand. Coffins were deposited on the ground by frightened cartmen, who promptly fled the scene, leaving the corpses to rot in the hot sun. By the second day, the bodies ballooned up large enough to burst open the coffins, allowing the putrid remains to spill out onto the ground, ghoulish reminders of what awaited those unfortunate enough to succumb to the disease.

Even so, vendors set up stands around the cemeteries, where they sold ice cream to combat the heat, brushes and mops to help clean up the oozing corpses, and sugar-filled candies to keep the children in high spirits, resembling modern-day concessions at rock concerts and football games as they made money off the suffering of others. The carnival atmosphere on the streets soon turned to chaos as the temperature dropped and the rains moved in, pummeling the city with a constant drizzle for ten days, sending residents behind closed windows to huddle beneath woolen blankets. When the sun finally emerged, it once again baked the streets with an intense, white heat that made the continuing stench even more offensive because of the humidity.

By the end of August, everyone who could afford to leave New Orleans had done so, but the exodus had no effect on the death toll, which, in some weeks, reached fifteen hundred. With the arrival of September, spirits improved because, even if no one knew what caused yellow fever or how it was transmitted, it was well understood that the disease did not thrive in cold weather. In mid-September, public health officials visited the temporary facilities that had been set up to handle the overflow from the hospitals, and they discovered that the number of patients had declined sharply.

With the epidemic severely curtailing commerce in the city over the summer, any activity that was not associated with caring for the sick, gathering bodies off the street, or burying the dead was deemed unnecessary, a prevailing public attitude that kept the streets relatively quiet. Newspaper reporters, surprised by the quietness of a downtown street, asked an elderly lady why her neighborhood was so still.

"Oh, sirs," she said. "It's very healthy here now."

"Healthy!" answered the reporters.

"Yes, sir," she said. "They be all dead—indeed, there be not fifteen left in the whole street."[6]

Once the disease was perceived to be winding down, newspapers once again declared New Orleans to be the most wonderful city in the world. On October 13, the health board declared that yellow fever "ceased to exist as an epidemic." Responding to that announcement, one newspaper editor gushed, "New Orleans is now perfectly healthy, and our absent citizens, whether acclimated or not, may return to the city with perfect safety."

Estimates of the death toll in New Orleans' 1853 epidemic vary from seventy-eight hundred to eleven thousand, making it the most deadly yellow fever epidemic to date in American history. Unlike the Philadelphia epidemic of 1793, which resulted in considerable debate among physicians about the treatment and transmission of the disease, the New Orleans epidemic left the American medical community baffled. They knew the symptoms; they knew that they would lose about half of the patients they treated; and they knew that the disease would run its course with the arrival of cold weather, but other than that they had little idea about the cause of the disease. Their research and note-taking would later prove invaluable to future generations of researchers, but they were unable to use that information to their own advantage. The most important lessons they learned were related to the day-to-day treatment of patients. The bloodletting and purging techniques advocated by Dr. Benjamin Rush were largely discounted, and the pre-epidemic attitude among physicians that massive doses of strong medications were essential for a full recovery from yellow fever was found to be without merit. Patients lived or died without apparent correlation with the treatment prescribed. Physicians did not advertise this discovery, but they lived with it on a daily basis, knowing that survival was based more on luck, or God's will, than on anything they could devise in the way of a treatment.

By the end of November, New Orleans had returned to normal in many respects, despite the appearance of Asiatic cholera. One of the city's most prominent physicians died of the disease, an event that fueled rumors of an epidemic. For a while, it appeared the city was headed for yet another nightmarish experience, with more than six hundred deaths attributed to the disease by year's end. As part of the city's public relations campaign to attract new business and visitors to the city, the mayor proclaimed: "I deem it my duty to state, for the information of persons abroad, that the health of our city was never better, and that visitors may come to New Orleans with impunity."

*   *   *

New Orleans residents who took a deep breath after living through the 1853 yellow fever epidemic were devastated the following year to find themselves going through yet another summer of hell. In 1854, 2,425 residents died of the disease. The following summer was even worse, with 2,670 deaths. The summers of 1856 and 1857 were relatively mild from a yellow fever standpoint, with a total of only 274 deaths, but the disease roared back in 1857, the year of the city's first Mardi Gras parade, claiming almost five thousand lives. No doubt the late afternoon and early evening parades contributed heavily to the death toll; since no one of that era knew what caused the disease, the outdoor celebrations were enjoyed amid a sort of ignorant bliss.

By the time the Civil War broke out in 1861, New Orleans, with a population of nearly 170,000, was the largest city in the South and the fifth-largest city in the United States, dual distinctions that quickly made it a target for invasion by federal troops. After only one year as a Confederate port, New Orleans was surrounded by Admiral David Farragut, a Tennessee-born naval officer who had begun his career in New Orleans.

Capturing the city did not require a major effort. Farragut encircled the city with gunboats and threatened to blast it to pieces with cannons if a quick surrender was not forthcoming. Within days, General Benjamin Butler entered the city with troops and took command. New Orleans spent the remainder of the war under occupation, a fact of life that the city's female population found particularly disagreeable. They wore Confederate emblems on their dresses to show their support of the cause, and they verbally taunted Union soldiers at every opportunity and hurled objects at them from balconies. Their behavior was tolerated until the day an irate woman emptied her chamber pot from her balcony onto the balding head of General Butler, an act that prompted the military to issue Order Number 28, which vowed to henceforth treat New Orleans' gentler sex as women "of the town plying their trade."

The order was greeted with indignation around the world, but Butler, who apparently never got over the chamber pot incident, refused to rescind the order, noting that it dramatically reduced the number of insults that soldiers had to endure while in New Orleans. Interestingly, during the four-year occupation, the city had only a total of eleven yellow fever cases. That was a cause of great distress to Southerners because they had hoped, indeed prayed, that yellow fever would conquer the Union army. Butler subsequently wrote in his memoir that he received reports that prayers were offered on a regular basis in city churches with the expectation that God would inflict an epidemic upon the invaders, especially "Beast" Butler, as he was then called by the gentler sex.

During Reconstruction (1865–1877), New Orleans struggled to regain its status as a major port and cultural center, a goal that was complicated by racial tension as activist white residents squandered their energies on blocking economic and political advancement among the city's African American population.

Reconstruction offered new opportunities to blacks who poured into the city during its occupation from all parts of the South. Many of them remained in the city to build a more democratic society. Not long after the war, the black-owned New Orleans *Tribune* proclaimed: "We wish to be respected and treated as men—not as Africans or Negroes or colored people, but as Americans and American citizens."

Blacks made progress by integrating public facilities, creating situations in which blacks sat in classrooms alongside whites. Blocked from sitting wherever they liked at the French Opera House, blacks sued for that right—and won. In 1874 a newspaper editor acknowledged the changes taking place in the city by noting: "In our midst the civil and public rights of the colored race [are] more fully realized than has been the case in any other southern city."[7]

During that time, yellow fever was little more than an annual nuisance, except in 1867, when the only epidemic of that period claimed 3,107 lives. There was a movement to provide public health officials with more money—and more political clout—to improve sanitary conditions in the city in the hopes of more effectively controlling future epidemics, but those efforts were stifled by the politics of Reconstruction. African Americans perceived the disease to be more of a white problem, with some justification, and they were slow to show support for public health proposals. Of course, those attitudes were not specific to New Orleans. One South Carolina physician, no doubt reflecting the opinion of medical workers across the South, lamented: "I despair of the State, in its present Africanized condition, spending money to improve health. Two-thirds of our Legislature would think such money thrown away."[8]

By the 1870s, public health was a major issue not just in New Orleans but throughout the South. Sanitation was the greatest weapon in the public health arsenal, but, as the years went by, quarantine gained in popularity because it fit the concept of yellow fever being a "foreign" threat. In time, they became opposing concepts. Sanitation advocates saw the disease as a local problem that was rooted in unhealthy living conditions; quarantine advocates were certain that the problem was the result of outside influences. Both sides, in their own way, were close to solving the yellow fever mystery, but being close didn't count for much, since the mortality rates for being close and being distant were exactly the same.

White businessmen were very much interested in public health because no single issue influenced their profits quite so much. People did business in New Orleans—or refused to do business—based on their perception of whether it was a safe place to visit. In the years following the end of the Civil War, tourists were hesitant to visit New Orleans, and shippers sometimes were reluctant to use the port.

When federal troops left New Orleans in 1877, it opened the door for white businessmen to regain power and create an agenda that elevated business issues over social issues. Blacks lost many of the gains they made during Reconstruction, but the economy improved dramatically, and New Orleans soon had cotton exports that neared pre–Civil War levels. Businessmen wasted no time becoming active in politics, and they soon had control of local government at all levels.

Throughout the 1870s, New Orleans businessmen opposed the concept of quarantine because they felt it brought business to a slow trickle during the summer months. W. C. Raymond, a prominent businessman, expressed the views of the new ruling class when he told the *Picayune* in the fall of 1878 that he was in favor of "no quarantine and taking our chances."

The problem that New Orleans businessmen faced was that decisions about quarantines were the responsibility of the

Louisiana State Board of Health, which oversaw quarantines not only in New Orleans but across the entire lower Mississippi Valley. In 1873 the New Orleans Chamber of Commerce, a body controlled by the city's business community, petitioned the federal government to assume control of the quarantine issue. For five years, pressure was put on Southern congressmen to obtain the enactment of legislation that would strip the state agency of its quarantine power, the idea being that federal control would give businessmen a better opportunity to influence the timing and duration of the quarantines.

Finally, on April 29, 1878, President Rutherford B. Hayes signed the Quarantine Act of 1878, which placed quarantines under the control of the surgeon general of the US Marine Hospital Service. However, the new law was not exactly the one requested by New Orleans businessmen because it prohibited federal infringement on the prerogatives of state and local health authorities. That left quarantine controls firmly in the hands of Samuel P. Choppin, president of the Louisiana State Board of Health. Choppin, who had served during the Civil War as medical inspector general of the Confederate Army, was highly regarded as a physician, and was a firm believer in the need for quarantines to control the spread of yellow fever.

The health board's frontline operation was the Mississippi Quarantine Station, located seventy miles south of New Orleans. From January through April, more than five hundred ships cleared the quarantine station.[9] Since there were reports of yellow fever that year in Brazil and Cuba, Choppin ordered the quarantine station to detain all boats from those ports for inspection and fumigation. The latter procedure was accomplished by burning pots of sulfur in the holds and by flushing the bilges with carbolic acid. If illness was detected in a crewman, he was immediately hospitalized at the station infirmary for observation.

Perhaps thinking that fumigation might damage the cargo, Choppin allowed ships carrying fruit to proceed into New Orleans without inspection. Oddly, he did not order inspections of all ships until mid-May. As a result, hundreds of ships docked in New Orleans in April and early May without inspection. It was also a time during which hundreds of Cuban refugees, fleeing their homeland, where civil war and yellow fever had resulted in many deaths, made their way into the city without being detained by authorities. It was during that period that the *Emily B. Souder* docked at the quarantine station. Three days out of Havana, it had arrived by way of Key West. When the station officer boarded the ship, he was met on the gangplank by the captain, who informed the officer that he had a crewman who was sick with fever.

After examining the crewman, the station officer diagnosed his illness as malaria and ordered him confined to the station infirmary. The remaining twenty-seven crewmen and nine passengers were examined and found to be in good health. Once the ship underwent fumigation procedures under the supervision of the station officer, it was allowed to enter New Orleans, where the captain presented his papers to custom officials and then docked at the foot of Calliope Street. Later that night, the captain became ill and was transported by a physician to the home of a mulatto nurse on Claiborne Street, where he was put to bed and provided with medication. When the physician returned the following morning to visit the captain, he discovered that he had taken a turn for the worse. The doctor changed the captain's medication and left instructions with the nurse for his treatment. The following day, the captain went into convulsions and died.

When questioned by reporters about the man's death, the attending physician attributed it to "intermittent bilious fever." By that time, another crewman had died aboard the ship. His body was sent to the morgue, where an autopsy was performed. The man was found to have yellow skin and a discolored liver that was noted to have "fatty degeneration." Orders were given to sprinkle carbolic acid around the two victims' lodgings. Within a week, the board of health sent a medical officer to investigate the deaths, which were then determined to be caused by yellow fever.

From the last week in May to the middle of July, customs officials recorded the arrival of eighteen ships from Cuba and another fifteen from other potentially infected ports.[10] No sooner had the *Emily B. Souder* left New Orleans than its berth was taken by the steamer *Charlie B. Woods*. After docking, the ship's captain and engineer, who lived in neighboring houses on Constance Street, joined their families for the duration of the layover. Two weeks later, one of their neighbors became ill with what was diagnosed by a Creole practitioner as malaria.

During that time, every member of the captain's and engineer's families became ill with a fever and then recovered. It was not until a physician was summoned to the neighborhood to treat a sick child that yellow fever was suspected. The physician reported the case to the board of health, but, after meeting with Dr. Choppin, the physician changed his diagnosis to malaria. That same day, the child died, after suffering from black vomit and convulsions. It was not until July 24 that the Louisiana State Board of Health made a public announcement that fourteen cases of yellow fever had been diagnosed in New Orleans. The acknowledgment of the presence of the disease was disquieting enough, but what sent everyone into a panic was news that most of the cases and deaths were among young children in a "good" section of town. This challenged two firmly held beliefs: the first being that children born in the city had acquired immunity to the disease from birth—and the second being that good sanitation was a preventative to the disease.

Once newspapers started publishing stories of new yellow fever cases, the panic was so overwhelming that an estimated 40,000 residents fled the city almost overnight, leaving behind about 170,000 people who had nowhere to go. All the ships and trains leaving the city were filled to capacity as terror-stricken families fled north, where they were not always warmly greeted, especially if they showed signs of any kind of illness. In some instances, the refugees were forcibly driven out of town by shotgun-toting vigilantes and threatened with death if they returned. Within days, New Orleans was quarantined by the state of Texas and by individual cities such as Mobile, Alabama, in an effort to keep the disease from spreading. However, not all communities were hostile to the refugees. Wrote one observer: "To the general rule, Louisville, Kentucky was a most noble exception: she opened her doors to all our refugees, her hospitals to the sick and her purse to the needy."

By mid-July, it was obvious that yellow fever had returned to New Orleans with a vengeance, giving the city its third-worst epidemic in history. "How it originated is a matter of dispute," noted one writer. "Some maintain it was indigenous; others say it was imported here toward the end of May from the West Indies by the steamer *Emily B. Souder* and the germs remained latent until circumstances favored its development. Just a few days previously, our papers and people had been congratulating themselves on their being exempted from the intolerant heat which prostrated and killed hundreds of people in St. Louis and other western and northern cities. But scarcely did it become known that yellow fever had certainly made its appearance in our city than people began to leave it in the greatest fright and terror, so that the trains and boasts scarcely take away all who wanted to leave."

By the end of August, there were 3,111 reported cases of yellow fever in New Orleans, with the number of new cases approaching three hundred a day. Observed a newspaper reporter: "A spirit of general uneasiness is for the first time prevalent. There is not a shadow of hope that there will be an abatement this month. On the contrary, the speedy seizure of all unacclimated persons is the only prospect."[11]

As in all other yellow fever epidemics in the city, those most affected by the enormity of it all were the physicians, priests, and ministers who literally fought the battle from street to street, house to house. Physicians averaged one hundred visits every twenty-four hours, with ministers and priests often following in their wake to comfort the dying and their survivors. "This epidemic spared neither age nor sex, neither rich nor poor, neither white nor black, neither foreigners nor native born, neither cleanliness nor filth," wrote a diarist in the house annals of the Redemptorist community. "The conclusion to be drawn from all this is that yellow fever is a very treacherous and mysterious disease. The best and most candid physicians and nurses must admit that the yellow fever baffles all their science and skill."

Because the demand was so large, the state board of health soon ran out of the preferred disinfectant and recommended that the public use a mixture of turpentine and water, which it proclaimed would "thoroughly deodorize and disinfect any ordinary sink or cesspool." Everyone seemed to agree that yellow fever was caused by a germ, but physicians had not reached the point where they were confident that germs could exist anywhere but in the air, water, or food. As a result, the state health board focused most of its efforts on protecting the food and water supply. When it came to treatment, the board admitted that preventative medicines were ineffective, and it went no further than to recommend a dose of oil to clear the bowels, a hot footbath to induce sweating, and plenty of bed rest. Unimpressed with those stark recommendations, the public turned to unscrupulous doctors around the country who promised cures, by means of mail order, for yellow fever with their "patented" elixirs. Noted one skeptical newspaper: "Hundreds of quacks in different parts of the country are trying to introduce their medicines in yellow fever here. Let them come to New Orleans and try it on themselves."[12]

At the end of September, the New Orleans health board reported 9,385 yellow fever cases, with 2,845 deaths. When pressed about the accuracy of the figures, authorities admitted that they probably were far below actual numbers. Indeed, some observers said that the true numbers were twice the reported numbers. There was not necessarily a conspiracy to underreport cases. Since the only way the board had of acquiring figures was to require physicians, hospitals, hotels, ship captains, and others to report cases to them, many cases went unreported and many residents suffered in silence without medical care, which many stubbornly avoided because they considered it no more effective than voodoo.

With the arrival of fall, there was optimism that the disease would soon run its course and allow the city to return to normal. The health board's official report for October listed 13,083 cases and 3,929 deaths for the season. A short time later, those figures were reevaluated and increased to "not less than 27,000" sick and "not less than 4,600" dead. With the arrival of the first frost on November 2, the number of cases quickly dwindled, allowing the city health board to announce its "final" recommendations of the season: citizens were asked to fumigate their homes with burning sulfur, and businessmen were asked to open their buildings and their crated merchandise to the cold air. Inspired by the optimistic mood sweeping the city, the *New Orleans Picayune* wrote with unrestrained glee that "the political cauldron is boiling, the organ grinder and the tramp have reappeared, and New Orleans is once more herself again."[13]

Once the city was safely past the 1878 epidemic, leaders again turned their attention to prevention. The New Orleans Medical and Surgical Association, which represented the majority of physicians in the city, made a shocking announcement that caught civic and business leaders off guard: "In order that our own people and the people of this country (at large) may not be misled by our silence, thus taking it as an endorsement of these [quarantine] schemes as proposed, [we] deem it proper to come forward and enter our protest against such measures and to suggest such means as we believe can alone render New Orleans a healthy city and free it from epidemics of yellow fever." The association said that its membership was convinced that yellow fever was a specific disease that, whatever its origins, was now endemic to the city. Since quarantine had never proved itself as an adequate preventative, the association recommended that it be used sparingly in the future. A more effective preventative measure, argued the association, would be for the city to undertake better drainage techniques, including the construction of an underground sewer system and the development of a more efficient garbage disposal system. The association's report was a shot in the arm for businessmen, who all along had argued that what was bad for business was bad for the city as a whole.

In a marked departure from their previous isolationist attitudes, New Orleans businessmen, many of them among the city's social elite, pooled their resources to get more involved in community health issues. They formed an organization called the Auxiliary Sanitary Association of New Orleans to assist the city in its cleanup operations. Money was raised among the businessmen to pay the wages of ten new sanitary inspectors, to purchase garbage scows and carts, and to establish a flushing system to clean the streets. Making liberal use of its slogan, "Public Heath Is Public Wealth," the association looked forward to the day when yellow fever would cease to cripple the city's commercial and social development.

Yellow fever returned to New Orleans in 1879, but only nineteen deaths were recorded. Not until 1897, when the city had almost three hundred deaths, did the disease threaten again in a major way. New Orleans' last yellow fever epidemic occurred in 1905, when more than four hundred residents lost their lives to a disease that, by then, had ceased being a major factor in the city's growth and development.

In 1907 the federal government took over the Louisiana quarantine system, thus completing what New Orleans businessmen had proposed decades ago. By then the city had municipal utilities in place to provide water, sewer, and drainage services, rendering the Auxiliary Sanitary Association obsolete. The fact that public officials were correct to insist that quarantine was an effective means of preventing yellow fever, but incorrect in identifying the targets of the quarantine, thus making the quarantine totally ineffective, is one of the great ironies of the city's recovery. The same thing can be said for its sanitation efforts. Clean streets and proper sewerage removal did wonders for the overall health of the city, but their role in controlling yellow fever was important only to the degree that they removed stagnant water from city streets and neighborhoods and not because they removed disease-carrying germs. Sometimes success is just another word for blind luck.

CHAPTER THREE

memphis
almost disappears

In the late 1700s, when Spanish explorers arrived at what is now Memphis, the Chickasaw Indians traded them a strip of land along the Mississippi River for food, weapons, and brandy. They built a fort high atop the bluff, along with an Indian trading post, but they never had more than a token presence in that area. When Spain ceded the land to the United States in 1795, the fort was abandoned and occupied by American troops under the command of Captain Meriwether Lewis. After Lewis's departure, a new fort was built several miles downriver and named Fort Pickering, after then secretary of state Timothy Pickering.[1]

Not long after Meriwether Lewis left the original fort, his good work was recognized by President Thomas Jefferson, who made him his private secretary, a position that required him to live in the president's home, Monticello. After the Louisiana Purchase, Jefferson asked Congress to appoint Lewis to lead an expedition into the new territory. Excited by the challenge—and eager to leave his secretary's position—Lewis asked an old friend, William Clark, to co-command the expedition with him.

At the conclusion of a wildly successful expedition, which took two-and-a-half years to complete, President Jefferson and Congress appointed Lewis governor of the Louisiana Territory, a position that required him to live in St. Louis, where he handled all government affairs in the territory and settled claims among Indian agents. Two years later, in 1809, Lewis was on his way to Washington, DC, to answer charges that he had misappropriated funds when he stopped at Fort Pickering. His plan was to travel by riverboat from Fort Pickering to New Orleans, where he could board a ship bound for the East Coast by way of the Florida Keys.

When Lewis stepped off the boat, he did not seem to be himself. The fort's commander noticed that Lewis was jaundiced, displayed indications of a high fever, and wobbled when he walked. He later described Lewis as "deranged." Upon his arrival, Lewis was advised not to proceed to New Orleans. Hostilities had broken out with the British, and there were reports that ships headed out of New Orleans were being seized by the British, who mistreated American passengers. Faced with that prospect, Lewis decided to take an overland route to Washington. He sent a letter to then president James Madison, stating his change in plans: "Providing my health permits, no time shall be lost in reaching Washington."

Lewis rested at the fort for two weeks and then set out for Nashville on horseback, a journey that took him across Chickasaw land to the Natchez Trace, a five-hundred-mile trail that stretched from Natchez to Nashville. It was there that the still-ailing thirty-five-year-old died in mysterious circumstances of gunshot wounds, the origins of which have never been determined. In all likelihood, Lewis was suffering from yellow fever at the time of his death. St. Louis, a city known for its swamps, had been subjected to yellow fever outbreaks ever since the Philadelphia epidemic of 1793. The fact that Lewis was traveling in September—traditionally a month of high activity for yellow fever—and possessed its major symptoms gives credence to the possibility that he had the disease and gave Memphis its first exposure.

Yellow fever was not the only danger lurking in the shadows of the bluff. In December 1811, two years after Lewis's visit to the fort, a Scottish scientist named John Bradbury was asleep on a riverboat about one hundred miles downstream from New Madrid, a small settlement south of where the Ohio River empties into the Mississippi River. Awakened by a "tremendous noise," he roused himself just in time to feel the boat lift into the air and then slap back down against the water. When he ran out onto the deck, he saw that "all nature seemed running into chaos." The night was filled with the terrifying sounds of falling timber, the screech of waterfowl, and the thunder of falling timber as huge chunks of the riverbank collapsed into the river.

Bradbury counted twenty-seven shocks. At sunrise, he was greeted by a raging river covered with foam and swirling debris. Ghost ships floated past, their crews nowhere to be seen. The earthquake that Bradbury survived was the greatest in American history. Centered at New Madrid, Missouri, it leveled that small town and then sent aftershocks that rumbled south, past Memphis to New Orleans, north to Detroit, and east to New England. Pavement was cracked as far away as Richmond and Washington. "The waters of the river gathered up like a mountain, fifteen to twenty feet perpendicularly, then receding within its banks with such violence that it took whole groves of cottonwoods which edged its borders," wrote Eliza Bryan, a New Madrid resident who survived the quake. "Fissures in the earth vomited forth sand and water, some closing again immediately."

A letter published in the *Lexington Reporter* told of "a most tremendous noise, while the house danced about and seemed as if it would fall on our heads. . . . At the time of this shock, the heavens were very clear and serene, not a breath of air stirring; but in five minutes it became very dark, and a vapour which seemed to impregnate the atmosphere, had a disagreeable smell, and produced a difficulty of respiration."

The earthquake of 1811 was a catastrophic event that would have leveled the Memphis settlement if there had been any buildings there large enough to be damaged. It would take many years for scientists to understand that New Madrid sits atop a three-thousand-foot-deep fault that cuts through five states along the Mississippi River. "New Madrid is the world's most spectacular example of liquefaction," said geologist Karl Mueller in a 1999 interview. "When you take a fine-grained, saturated sediment like mud or silt and you shake it during an earthquake, it turns to the consistency of Jell-o. If you have a building that is sitting on top of Jell-o, the building falls down. The scary part about New Madrid is that . . . we see liquefaction all over the place there."[2]

One of the side effects of liquefaction is the creation of pockets in the earth. The largest pocket created by the 1811 earthquake is the thirteen-thousand-acre Lake Reelfoot, located north of Memphis. Thousands of smaller pockets were created around Memphis, all of which became basins for stagnant water, the best friend that yellow fever could possibly have. The disease was a constant threat to the area, from the earliest days on, but not until 1828 was there a documented yellow fever epidemic. There were 650 recorded cases and 150 deaths, a major disaster in a community the size of Memphis.

Despite the threats from yellow fever and earthquakes, Memphis grew and prospered. At the site of the original fort in Memphis, white settlers built a frontier community that stubbornly clung to the bluff, an island of immigrant optimism in a sea of Chickasaw culture that had defined the area for more than ten thousand years. The settlers, who numbered no more than fifty, were afforded a degree of permanency when North Carolina, which then claimed ownership to what would later become the state of Tennessee, sold sixteen square miles of land around the fort to two speculators who envisioned a great city.

One of the surveyors who laid out the boundaries for the city was Marcus B. Winchester, the son of James Winchester, who had been instrumental in obtaining the land for the original speculators, one of whom later sold half of his land to Judge John Overton, who sold half to future president Andrew Jackson, who sold half to the Winchesters. When the time name to name the new city, its three owners—the Winchesters, Judge Overton, and Andrew Jackson, none of whom ever lived in Memphis—looked to the ancient Middle East and took the name of an Egyptian town located on the Nile River near the Abu Sir Pyramids. The Egyptian Memphis was founded around 3100 BCE and was a major trading center throughout the Hellenistic and early Roman periods and a target of Alexander the Great. It was abandoned following the 640 CE Arab conquest and allowed to disappear in the desert sand.[3]

What Memphis's founders saw in the name may never be known, for, unlike its cosmopolitan Egyptian predecessor, it was little more than a wide-open frontier outpost, a shantytown with muddy streets and rugged log cabins. From its official founding in 1819, it took more than twenty years for Memphis to establish itself as an important port, and, when recognition finally came, it was because of the export of cotton and the importation of slaves to work the plantations in the surrounding area.

By 1852, Memphis was the third most important port on the Mississippi, well on its way to becoming the fastest-growing city in America. Unfortunately, the city's emerging good fortune was based on the slave trade. For many years, slavery was prohibited in Tennessee, but, as the demand for slaves grew in the Mississippi Delta and elsewhere, slave dealers began operating in defiance of the law. Eventually, slavery became so lucrative in Memphis that the Tennessee legislature was persuaded to repeal the state's prohibition on slave trading.

As the African American population in Memphis increased (prior to 1860, only 17 percent of the residents were black), so did the legal restrictions against them, even though the free blacks in the city numbered fewer than fifty. A 10:00 PM curfew was imposed on blacks, with a promise that all violators would be arrested and taken to jail, where they would remain overnight. Free blacks were assessed a ten-dollar fine; if they did not have the money, they were forced to work for the city until the fine was paid. Slaves who violated the curfew were given ten lashes across the back and sent home, with a two-dollar fine imposed on their owners.

As Memphis experienced an economic boom throughout the 1840s and 1850s, the population increased dramatically, with German and Irish immigrants playing a significant role in that success. From a population of eighteen hundred in 1840, the city exploded to more than twenty-two thousand people in 1858. Banks and office buildings were constructed, along with a luxury hotel, the Gayoso House, that offered flush toilets and hot showers at a time when such conveniences were almost nonexistent in private residences. The only thing that slowed the city's momentum, even slightly, was the 1855 yellow fever epidemic, which killed 220 Memphians. Not only did the epidemic not prompt a panic, it made residents feel superior to their business competitors in New Orleans, where yellow fever death tolls each year were often ten to twenty times as high as those in Memphis.

*   *   *

In the 1860 presidential election, 90 percent of Memphis voters sided with pro-Union candidates John Bell and Stephen A. Douglas, so there were questions in some people's minds whether the city would go with the South or remain in the Union—at least, until the siege and fall of South Carolina's Fort Sumter, which tipped the balance in favor of the fledgling Confederacy.

Confederate general Leonidas Polk, a former Episcopal bishop, set up his headquarters at the Gayoso House and began a recruiting effort that resulted in nearly four thousand men enlisting at the first call, an extraordinary burst of patriotism that made headlines across the country since Memphis had a population of only twenty-two thousand, 17 percent of whom were African Americans. Do the math, and you will see that almost half the white men in Memphis, from infancy to old age, volunteered to fight.

Once the war began in earnest, Memphians were confident that the Union would be defeated within a matter of months. Oddly, the city did very little to bolster its defenses, relying instead on positions taken upriver by Confederate forces—and by defenses established on the Cumberland and Tennessee rivers. That confidence was shattered by early 1862, when Tennessee's defenses began falling at an astonishing rate.

For months, Memphians prepared for an invasion, but when Union forces arrived, the assault came by river and not land. As the Union fleet, which was composed of five ironclads and nineteen rams, arrived to do battle with Memphis's ramshackle river fleet (eight converted steamboats), a reported ten thousand citizens assembled on the bluffs to watch the Yankees tuck tail and run. It didn't happen that way. The Union ships quickly overpowered the Confederate navy in a battle that lasted less than ninety minutes, at the end of which Union officers entered Memphis under a white flag and demanded its surrender. Later that day, the American flag was raised over the post office.

With Memphis firmly under Union control, General William T. Sherman arrived at Fort Pickering and expanded it into a two-mile-long fortification, large enough to accommodate ten thousand troops. It was the largest and most elaborate fortification of any city in the nation, other than Washington, DC. To build the fort, Sherman pressed about six thousand African Americans into forced labor, both slaves and free men, providing them food, clothing, shelter, and one pound of chewing tobacco each month.

Despite harsh treatment at the hands of the "liberation" army, more than fifteen thousand African Americans poured into Memphis from the surrounding areas, giving the city, for the first time in its history, a majority black population. In 1864 more than seven thousand African Americans, almost all of them former slaves, enlisted in the Union army and saw combat service against their masters in the Confederate army.

By the end of the war, Memphis was a shambles of its former

self, not physically, because nothing more aggressive than small-arms fire ever took place in the city, but, rather, socially and economically. The city was poorly equipped to handle the thousands of African Americans who arrived with no money and no place to live. As a result, shantytowns sprang up along the outskirts of the city, where unemployed African Americans huddled together in tents or poorly built shelters and existed on meager government rations, living in deplorable conditions in neighborhoods that had little or no provisions for sanitation or the proper drainage of rainwater.

Under the terms of Reconstruction, Confederate veterans were prohibited from voting or running for elective office. Since women were still more than half a century away from obtaining the right to vote, the voting pool comprised white men who never served in the Confederacy, carpetbaggers from the North, immigrants from Ireland, and black men who went directly from slavery into the voting booth.

Reconstruction provided African Americans with political power but did nothing to give them economic power. Frustrations built for months and erupted into violence in May 1866 with a race riot that lasted for three days. Forty-six persons died, forty-four of them African American, and seventy-five persons were wounded. When the smoke cleared, four churches were burned, along with twelve schools and almost one hundred homes. White troops were sent from Nashville to bring order, and the city was placed under martial law.

A United States Army inquiry determined that African Americans under the influence of alcohol started the riot because of hard feelings over competition with poor Irish immigrants for low-paying jobs, but whites were blamed for escalating the fighting and prolonging it beyond the point of reason to its deadly conclusion.

Memphis limped along into 1867, struggling to build a new society. It was into that atmosphere that yellow fever made its insidious return, with an epidemic that claimed 595 lives and made an already fearful city even more apprehensive about the future. The records of one physician's office are revealing: Of 256 cases treated by the physician, 193 recovered and 63 died, providing him with a higher success rate for treatment than most physicians of that era.

Over the next few years, Memphis became the center of Ku Klux Klan activity in the area, with former Confederate general Nathan Bedford Forrest as its Grand Wizard, but white extremists actually had little impact on Reconstruction. On the contrary, militant black leaders, such as Ed Shaw, emerged to lead African Americans to unprecedented victories in the voting booth. Blacks won two city council seats in 1872 and four seats in 1873. Shaw was soon elected wharfmaster, the highest-paying office in local government.[4] During that time, Jefferson Davis, the former president of the Confederacy, relocated to Memphis with his family, where he worked as the head of an insurance firm, apparently unconcerned about black political gains.

Outside of the war, Memphis's biggest challenge to date occurred in 1873. On the tenth of August, the towboat *Bee* docked at the foot of Market Street in a neighborhood called "Happy Hollow," a derisive term that was used to show contempt for the poor people who lived on boats in the placid backwash of the river. The *Bee* had made its way to Memphis from New Orleans on its way to St. Louis.

The boat remained for several hours, long enough to take on fresh meat and other supplies and to allow the captain to receive medical treatment. The boat left that afternoon and proceeded upriver only to run into trouble the following night, about ninety miles north of Memphis, when the ship's captain suddenly died. His body was loaded onto the steamer *Fulton City* and returned to Memphis, where, after lying out on the wharf for several hours in full view of passersby, it was prepared for express shipment to St. Louis (a process that involved packing the body with charcoal and plenty of ice). While the *Fulton City* was docked in Memphis, a jaundiced passenger left the boat and sat outside one of the cabins located near the water. The owner of the house, an Irishman named Riley, took him in, but the man died the next day. Doctors attributed his condition to bilious fever, a general term used to label jaundiced patients whose cause of disease could not be determined. A second passenger, an elderly man who was on his way to Alabama after visiting Texas, left the boat and spent the night at a hotel, only to die the next morning. Later, it was learned that he had passed through Shreveport, which was known to be in the midst of a yellow fever epidemic, on his way to New Orleans, where he boarded the *Bee.*

"The disease began to spread from the point where the boat landed, and it seems that the fatal infection came from the boat rather than those who were landed and left to die," concluded one report. "The first victim known was a young man who had assisted the poor fellow off who died at Riley's house. Then Riley himself was stricken down and soon died; after that about two persons died per day for two weeks but without exciting any alarm. If any of the doctors discovered that it was yellow fever, they prudently kept their own counsels, as it was at that time, and even later, a high crime to tell any truth that would drive off trade or 'ruin the city.'"[5]

By September 1, the disease had spread from its initial point of entry about three hundred yards to the top of the bluff, making its way into the downtown area, where a well-known steamboat man died of a fever at his hotel, followed within days by the death of his wife. Not until September 14 did the Memphis Board of Health acknowledge that the city was having a yellow fever epidemic.

Not happy with the health board's decision was the Memphis *Appeal*, which wrote:

We regret the manner in which the board of health yesterday published a declaration that there is yellow fever in Memphis. The declaration did make it clear, however, that there is no epidemic and that the yellow fever is confirmed to one locality, in the northeastern part of the city. But we fear the intention of the board. No doubt the resolution will be widely misunderstood by our people and will be taken to mean that the dread disease is here in epidemic form. Only five death certificates were issued this week with yellow fever named as the cause of death. The resolution of the board of health stated that there were "about 30." On behalf of our mercantile interests, which have already suffered much from epidemic scares, we urge our citizens to remain calm. There is no yellow fever epidemic. When there is, *The Appeal* will say so.[6]

At the urging of citizens, the city council appropriated $10,000 to the Howard Association of Memphis, a relief organization. Before the month was out, the Howards converted a house into a hospital for the care of yellow fever patients. Physicians who specialized in yellow fever were brought in from Louisville, Kentucky, and Mobile, Alabama, and nurses were recruited throughout the South. Of the seventy nurses who answered the call, twenty died of the fever.

Interestingly, there were no accounts of African Americans coming down with the disease, a fact that clearly inflamed the passions of racists who used the issue to promote prejudice. Consider this from a minister, the Rev. S. A. Quinn: "One early morning of the ninth of October 1873, near the corners of Main and Jackson streets, a group of half terrified Negroes surrounded the carcass of a mule that lay stretched in the middle of the street. . . . At last, a Negro whose cropped, but frosted hair bespoke the winter of 'three score and ten,' in the capacity of a spokesman said: 'Colored sisters and brothers: when de Feber takes de mule, de Nigger han't got no show.' This process of reasoning although contrary to Christian cosmogony, did not militate against the theories of Darwin, who acknowledged no distinction between animal protoplasms. In fact, the colored spokesman, according to the latter writer, made a logical deduction, predicting no escape for his people."[7]

City officials estimated that the disease advanced through the city at the rate of about one block a week. As one report concluded:

> It was remarkably fatal and for some weeks baffled medical treatment. . . . Many died after a very short illness, varying from two to four days. The physicians were not agreed at first as to the nature of the disease. . . . We will say, however, that the physicians, in their noble efforts to alleviate suffering, finally became quite successful in their management of the fever, and that many of the very worst cases were brought through to a safe issue. . . . The people were stunned, demoralized, and knew not what to do. . . . It was a time of great public peril, and never was a leader so badly needed; someone to assure the people, and set on foot the proper measures of relief. While hundreds of people were leaving on every train, thousands could not get away. They could not shut up their houses, their shops and stores, as many did not have the means to take their large families to the country, even if assured of free board when they got there.

By the time the epidemic had run its course—the first frost came on October 7—about five thousand cases were reported, with more than two thousand deaths. The disease so ravaged the city that a special census undertaken three years later revealed that the city's population had increased by only four persons since 1870. At that time, of course, no one knew what caused yellow fever, but since there was considerable filth and standing water in the city, elected officials determined that the disease was the result of noxious gases that rose from the filth. To combat the gases, they fired cannons to dispel the deadly gases they imagined hovering over the city. As terrifying as it was to those who lived through it, the 1873 epidemic was but a harbinger of much worse to come.

*   *   *

Five years after the 1873 epidemic, little had changed in Memphis. The rich got richer and the poor got poorer, as the city found itself mired in political and economic lethargy. Since few citizens had any money, there was no way for the city to raise enough tax revenues to make the sort of improvements that were needed to provide essential services. Pledges made at the end of the 1873 epidemic to clean up the trash and drain the standing water were never carried out and by 1878 little had changed in the city. Because of the filth, the city resembled an abandoned farmyard more than it did an important port city. The water supply, which came from wells or from a plant that was supposed to "purify" water from the river, was putrid, and the milk supply was even worse—a local newspaper reported an instance of a live minnow swimming about in a pail of milk that was offered for sale.

The winter and early spring of 1878 were cold and gray, with intermittent rain that fell in sheets. On those few days when the sun came out, spirits were lifted with visions of a better tomorrow, perhaps never so much as during the city's Mardi Gras celebration in early March. One of the participants that year was a young girl named Belle Wade, a sensitive girl who recorded her thoughts in a diary:

> Although it is "Mardi Gras" I am not able to go out and have got the sore throat so badly I don't know what to do—and a dreadful cold. Mr. Witzmann [a language teacher at Memphis High School who taught music on the side] did not come today. After we ate supper, we all went up town to see the "Memphis" procession, which was grand and magnificent. They represented Greece and Scandinavia. After we saw the procession on Main Street we went down to the bluff to see the fireworks, which were lovely. We then went back to Main Street to try to see the procession again, but the crowd was so great that we didn't succeed. I reckon this was the most beautiful day we have ever had on Mardi Gras.[8]

Three days later, on March 8, Belle wrote: "My cold is still no better. I took my music lesson this morning and Mr. Witzmann said he forgot it today but he was going to send me some cough medicine that would cure me right off. I told him I would never see that medicine. Tonight the bell rang and Melissa brought me a note and a package. I opened it and lo! It was candy. The note was from Mr. Witzmann. The candy is just splendid."

As early as May, word reached Memphis of a yellow fever outbreak in the West Indies, but the city ignored a quarantine request from the merchants. In early July, there were isolated reports of transients who died of illnesses that could have been yellow fever, but, since no blood tests existed at that time to determine whether an individual had yellow fever or some other disease that affected the liver, diagnosis depended entirely on a physician's analysis of the patient's symptoms. The physicians who cared for the transients were reluctant to diagnosis yellow fever for fear of starting a panic. After all, the patients could have died of infectious hepatitis, a disease that involves jaundice and fever.

The only real "test" that physicians had to diagnosis yellow fever was the thermometer. Wrote one Memphis physician in the 1870s: "The fever in cases which progressed regularly and favorable reached its greatest intensity within the first twenty-four hours of the attack, usually reaching 102 degrees and 103 degrees, after which it would decline about 1 degree, preserving this range for two days longer, and then slowly decline, passing off from the third to fifth day. In dangerous or fatal cases it would continue to rise to 104 degrees and higher, till the fourth day, after which it declines very rapidly for from one to two days, leaving the patient in a state of alarming or fatal prostration, death beginning at the heart. In other cases, just before death, it would rise to 105 degrees, 106 degrees, and above this height."

That same physician challenged the popular medical assumption that black vomit was the one true sign of impending death. "Suppressed urine was the fatal sign, not the black vomit," he wrote, "whereas a larger proportion of cases of black vomit than usual recovered where the urinary secretion was not suspended." (The physician was correct to link urinary problems to liver failure, a link that was not understood until many years later). The physician also noted that the disease created additional problems for women: "The disease was very fatal to pregnant women, causing frequent abortions, and resulting in death from exhaustion."

On July 26 word reached Memphis that the *John Porter*, the towboat that had been publicized as the starting point for the yellow fever epidemic in New Orleans, was headed for Memphis after dropping off two "sunstroke" cases at Vicksburg that later proved to be yellow fever. That evening, appearing before the city health board, the mayor said, "That it exists in New Orleans at this time cannot now be doubted, and that it may be brought here by river communication is equally unquestioned. We owe it to the public to diminish the possibilities of the visitation of this dreadful scourge, and so I must urge upon you the adoption of any means to secure this end." The next day, quarantine stations were set up on the two railroads that entered the city to identify feverish individuals who traveled by land and on a nearby island in the Mississippi River to evaluate ships such as the *John Porter*. Freight trains entering Memphis were ordered to unload their cargoes several miles outside the city for ten days' detainment and disinfection, and all freight originating in New Orleans or Vicksburg was ordered to be returned to its port of origin. Any suspicious-looking passengers were escorted to the city hospital for observation.

Two weeks before the quarantine went into effect, isolated reports of illness began circulating in the city. On July 15, Belle Wade wrote in her diary that her father was ill: "Papa came home feeling dreadfully today. I do hope he is not going to be sick," followed the next day with, "Papa came home sick again tonight. He says he has not been able to work since two o'clock. Am so sorry he is sick." Three days later she wrote: "Papa came home feeling worse than ever tonight. I am so sorry. I hope he will be better in the morning. As I didn't get home from Mrs. McKisick's until one o'clock I didn't practice but three hours so I have got an hour to make up. I took a music lesson this evening."

Belle's diary entries continued to paint a vivid picture of the hopes and fears of adult Memphians:

July 20, 1878

Papa was so sick this morning he had to stay home and send for the doctor which I think he should have done before. It is still very hot—some say they never knew such hot weather to last such a long time. I know I never felt such hot weather in all my life. I went over to the church with Susie today when she went to practice and it was so hot over there it gave me a dreadful headache so I didn't practice but three hours again today. I think I will make up a quarter of an hour each day.

July 21, 1878

I went to Sunday school and church this morning. Papa felt too badly, so we were put in Mrs. Camel's class. It is still dreadfully warm and so dusty. I do wonder how much longer this weather will last. Mr. John Law preached this morning. As it was so warm we didn't have any preaching tonight.

July 22, 1878

Papa didn't feel any better this morning but went uptown: he had to take his medicine at nine o'clock, so I took it up to him, but when I got up there, he had gone home feeling worse. I am so sorry he is sick. He sent for the doctor as soon as he got home, and I think he is a little better this evening. It has been delightful today. It has turned so much cooler, but still very dusty.

July 26, 1878

We are very much afraid we will have the yellow fever here. They have it at New Orleans. I do hope we won't.

*   *   *

With fears of an epidemic dominating conversations on the street, a local newspaper attempted to defuse the situation by denying the obvious: "There is considerable uneasiness in Memphis. Frightened people repeat frightful stories of cases all over the city, and men who ought to have better sense, and more manliness, are giving currency to wild reports. . . . As a matter of fact Memphis was never in summer freer from disease of all kinds than now."[9]

On August 12, 1878, public apprehension about an epidemic surged with word from Grenada, Mississippi, about one hundred miles south of Memphis, that the town was in the midst of a yellow fever epidemic. There were reports that the sheriff and all the city officers had fled the town and that the banks had closed their doors, along with most of the merchants, actions that sent the citizens into a panic.

The following day, the Memphis board of health posted armed guards at all stations leading into the city from Grenada. In the minds of many, it was a case of too little, too late. Before the day was over, the Memphis health board announced that the city had its first confirmed yellow fever death—Kate Bionda, the owner of a snack shop located on Front Street, near the river. That news was all Memphians needed to work themselves up into a full-fledged panic.

Within four days of that announcement, more than half the city's forty thousand residents had fled to the countryside, where for a two-hundred-mile radius they were greeted by club-toting vigilantes determined to prevent them from entering their communities. The *Memphis Appeal* put the exodus in perspective:

"Stores and offices were hastily closed. . . . Men, women and children poured out of the city by every possible avenue of escape. . . . Out by every possible conveyance—by hack, by carriages, buggies, wagons, furniture vans, and street drays; and by the railroads. . . . The stream of passengers seemed to be endless and they seemed to be as mad as they were many. The ordinary courtesies of life were ignored; politeness gave way to selfishness and the desire for personal safety broke through all the social amenities."

The day of the announcement, Belle Wade wrote in her diary: "There is great excitement here about the 'Yellow Fever.' We heard it is here, but do not know whether it is so or not. Oh! I do hope it is not." Then, the following day, she wrote: "Yellow Fever is here sure enough. A man and woman have died of it, and several other cases are reported. Everybody is going away nearly. I heard a thousand people went night before last. It is impossible for us to go. I practiced four hours today. There are eight cases of Yellow Fever here."

Belle tried to be brave about her family's prospects, but it was difficult under the circumstances: "There are twenty-two cases of Yellow Fever here, so it was reported in the morning paper. I hope and pray none of us will have it. . . . We did have such a time killing time today. We were so lonely. We named the corners of the room. Last night the gentlemen teased us a great deal about it. They wanted us to tell them who we named them, but we wouldn't do it. There were 40 new cases of Yellow Fever yesterday. . . . There is nobody left here now but Lily, myself and some colored people. We started to take a walk this morning, but we saw a snake and I came very near stepping on it. We were so frightened we came back home."

With the death of Kate Bionda, health officials descended upon the location where she operated her business and cordoned the entire block off and posted police officers along the perimeter. The site was then washed with bucket after bucket of coal oil and carbolic acid, staining the sidewalks black and filling the air with the stifling odor of lime and tar. After the health officer inspected the business, the *Avalanche* reported: "A bad dwelling place, redolent with the odor of fish. There the woman, an habitual and very hard drinker, lived, right in among the fumes of her food and its debris and its trash. A boatman from New Orleans, had he carried in his clothes to that spot the smallest amount of contagion, it would have found a soil in which the seed of disease could not but germinate."

Most of the twenty thousand residents who remained in the city were African Americans, many of them former slaves. They stayed throughout the epidemic, supplying the majority of the three thousand nurses who cared for the sick and dying. They distributed the supplies that poured in from all over the country, and they collected and buried thousands of corpses. When the white police force fled the city in fear, African Americans formed two militia companies that patrolled the streets to keep the peace and to prevent looting.

Irish immigrants made up another large block of those who remained, as did more than three thousand Jews, some of whom fled to St. Louis and Cincinnati. Noting the Jews who stayed behind, the Hebrew Hospital Association observed that "the suffering among our co-religionists was as great as any. The bulk of them were poor and destitute and unable to reach places of safety . . . [when] the fever reached its zenith. . . . To our utter dismay we found every avenue leading to the city densely packed with Jewish families, and with few exceptions did any escape the force of the fever."[10] Nathan Menken, the founder, with his brothers, of Menken Brothers Dry Goods, certainly had the money to leave the city, but he did not, electing to send only his wife and two children north. Instead, he got involved in relief efforts, using his position as president of the Hebrew Hospital Association to provide for the sick and dying. He worked day and night in that part of the city hit hardest by the epidemic, and he undoubtedly made a difference in the lives of many. Unfortunately, he contracted the disease himself, dying without ever again seeing his wife and children.

Special police details were sent throughout the city to look for the dead and dying and to encourage others to flee to the camps set up five miles outside the city. The *Avalanche* reported the experiences of one police detail that entered a tenement house off Commerce Street: "Upon the bed lay the living and the dead—a husband cold and stiff, a wife in the agony of dissolution. On the floor, tossing in delirium, were two children of this pair, and beside them their little cousins, two little girls, themselves sick. To complete the repulsiveness of the scene and give it a touch of disgusting horror, a drunken man and a drunken woman, parents of the little fever-baked girls, were reeling and cursing, and stumbling over the dying and the dead."[11]

Each day, the death escalated at a terrifying rate. On August 29, 140 new cases of yellow fever were reported, along with seventy deaths. A woman was found in a hut on Main Street, sitting in a chair, dead, with a dead child hanging by the nipple of her left breast. A second child was found lying on the floor on a pallet, but, before he could be removed to a hospital, he died on the spot. Health officers reported that the walls, floor, and everything in the room were covered with black vomit. The mother and children were buried in the same box. Not far away, on Poplar Street, the remains of an old woman were found lying on a piece of carpet. The festering flesh, which seemed to float in a soup of putrid water, was so decayed that health officials simply picked up the carpet, remains and all, and deposited it in a box that was buried in a potter's field.

A man riding a horse along the same street was so sickened by the stench coming from a building near the market house that he stopped and entered the building, breaking down the door of a first-floor room, where he discovered a dead body in an advanced stage of decomposition—the corpse of a barber. In a nearby building, nurses found two bodies in one room, three bodies in another room, and four bodies in a third room, so many that undertakers did not have time to bury them. When the undertaker complained and gave the health officer a hard time about his workload, a warrant was issued for his arrest. He got wind of it and eluded police officers, but an investigation revealed that he was storing yellow fever corpses in his stable on Union Street until a wagon load could be collected and transported to a potter's field.

The epidemic was like a rampaging river that knocked down everything in its path, casting men, women, and children into one horrific situation after another, an occurrence that made moments of grace difficult to find, though sometimes goodness did roam the landscape in a more or less random manner. Consider the young girl, some said she was beautiful beyond belief, who kept the registry of the dead at Elwood Cemetery at the request of her father, and she spent hours at a time tolling a bell that offered hope and encouragement to those who had not yet had occasion to visit the cemetery. She remained at her post, a courageous clerk, until she came down with the fever. Fortunately, she recovered and resumed her post, her constantly tolling bell the only one heard in the city.

There was romance associated with the death of Zach Oliver, a Memphis letter carrier. One day, while on his way home, he encountered a young Jewish woman named Phoebe Mendleson who had come into the city to inquire about letters she hoped to receive from her parents, who had fled north in the first days of the epidemic. Seeing that the woman was very ill, Oliver took her to his lodgings and rushed out to find a physician to care for her. By the time she recovered well enough to sit up, Oliver was stricken with the fever. Although in a weakened state from her own disease, she nursed her new friend, who lingered for a few days and then died in her arms.

A citizens' relief committeeman walked into a humble cottage in the southern part of the city, where he found two children ill, one weak and listless but evidently convalescing and the other tossing in burning fever. A woman dressed in black sat between the two children and was in the process of kissing the brow of the fevered one when the committeeman entered.

"Can't I send you a nurse, madam?" he asked.

"No sir," she answered, smiling. "I have brought one child through, and I shall bring the other."

"But you are worn out."

"Oh, no, sir—a kind Italian woman nearby comes in and helps me sometimes."

The woman refused the committeeman's help, confident that her love would prevail.[12]

*   *   *

Annie Cook, a beautiful girl of German descent, was not considered a pillar of Memphis society, though she often had intimate contact with the city's leading citizens. As the proprietor of a bordello named Mansion House that offered run-of-the-mill sex for fifty cents an hour—and more exotic experiences for an additional ten cents—she was pretty much a creature of the night, seldom coming into view as long as the sun was strong enough to cast shadows under her brightly painted eyes.

All that changed, however, with the arrival of the epidemic. She sent her girls away and opened up Mansion House to the sick and dying, venturing into the daylight to find those in pain. To everyone's surprise, she acted out the "prostitute with a heart of gold" myth, wrapping herself in aprons to nurse those most in need of tender loving care. As might be expected, she herself came down with the fever and died, her body buried in an unmarked grave not far from downtown.

Touched by her death was a Kentucky newspaper editor who had known the woman before she moved to Memphis, though in exactly what capacity he knew her he never disclosed. "Yesterday the wires whispered the news of her death," he wrote. "Poor, ill-starred, misguided woman! Whatever her sins may have been, she has laid them all down with her life, and may we not hope that her chances for her life of happiness 'up there' are secured by an earnest repentance and a self-sacrifice that cost her life. Mary Magdalen became the most devoted of His followers, and now that Annie Cook's life has ended in sacrifice for others, there is hope that it may be said to her, 'For as much as ye did it unto the least of these, ye did it also unto me.'"

By the middle of September, the epidemic was killing one hundred people each day, with hundreds of new cases appearing as quickly as the corpses were put underground. Interviewed many years later, Dr. Charles T. Davis, a survivor of the epidemic, told a newspaper reporter that the death wagons worked in pairs: "One wagon left the coffins and the other picked them up after they had been filled. Negroes did all that kind of work. They were practically immune to the fever. When one of them got it, you could bet that he was a mulatto."

When yellow fever first appeared in a household, Dr. Davis explained, a piece of yellow cardboard was placed near the door.

When the victim died, a black cardboard was placed beside the yellow one. The dimensions of the coffin needed were written on the black board with chalk. A man came by and took down the number of the house and the size of the coffin. . . . Well, after the black sign was put out, a coffin was delivered at the door. The corpse was placed in the box by relatives, along with a mixture of tar and acid. The lid was bolted on. Then the six-horse death wagon stopped outside. The melancholy cry, "Bring out your dead," came through the tightly shuttered windows. The coffin was placed on the porch and then piled on the wagon. Grave diggers worked in relays all the time. There were few services at the graves. Most of the coffins were just dumped in and the holes filled in. The nights were awful. Intense heat, the odor of the burning tar, the rattle of the death wagons and the eerie sound of a moaning city, praying, dying.[13]

A man who nursed a young girl, probably his niece, wrote of that experience to a relative who was in a place of safety. "Lucille died at ten o'clock Tuesday night, after such suffering as I hope never again to witness," he wrote. "Once or twice my nerve almost failed me, but I managed to stay. The poor girl's screams might be heard for half a square and at times I had to exert my utmost strength to hold her in bed. Jaundice was marked, the skin being a bright yellow hue: tongue and lips dark, cracked and blood oozing from the mouth and nose." As bad as that was, he continued, it was nothing compared to what followed. "To me, the most terrible and terrifying feature was the 'black vomit' which I never before witnessed. By Tuesday it was as black as ink and would be ejected with terrific force. I had my face and hands spattered but had to stand by and hold her. Well, it is too terrible to write any more about it."[14]

Memphians who could not or would not leave the city often wrote letters to family and friends who lived in safe locations, but they never knew when, or even if, their letters would be delivered, since the city's postal service was as ravaged by the disease as any other service or business. Every letter that made it out of the city bore a distinct postmark—five or six holes punched though the paper. The holes were made by a wooden paddle studded with nails. Postal workers dipped the paddle into a sulfur solution and then pounded the mail with the paddle in an attempt to fumigate the paper, leaving the telltale holes that let recipients know that their mail had been posted in a city in which yellow fever was raging. The decision as to whether the pocked envelopes should be opened, or buried in a deep hole, was left to the recipients

Some residents, like Belle Wade, sent letters to themselves in the form of diary entries, perhaps hopeful that someday others would receive their thoughts and reflect on their situation during the epidemic. At the end of August, Belle wrote: "I commenced a book Mrs. Baskin lent Susie [Belle's older sister] today and nearly finished it. The title was 'Edna Browning.' It is a splendid book. It rained a good while and very hard yesterday and has turned right cool. There were 140 new cases yesterday and seventy-three deaths." The following day, she wrote: "I finished my book today. It was very interesting. The fever is so bad the doctors haven't time to report the new cases." Belle attempted to instill a sense of normalcy in her situation by reading books and visiting friends to offset the horror that swirled all around her. Her diary entries for the next week were curious mixtures of youthful optimism and nightmarish fright:

September 2, 1878

Lily and I went to Mrs. Baskin's this evening to return some books. We had a very pleasant visit. When we came away Mrs. Baskin lent us each a book. There were 200 new cases during Saturday and today and 102 deaths. Mr. Boggs [Reverend William E. Boggs, pastor of the Second Presbyterian Church] is going to send his children away tomorrow.

September 3, 1878

I like my book so far very much. The title is "Ernest Linwood." Mr. B. P. Anderson died in Grenada yesterday of yellow fever. He has been there nursing the sick ever since it made its appearance there. Oh! How sorry I do feel for poor Katie. There were ninety deaths yesterday. The physicians haven't the time to report the new cases. It is so dreadfully warm.

September 4, 1878

I finished my book today. It was beautiful. There were 208 interments in the last twenty-four hours.

September 5, 1878

I went over to Mrs. Baskin's this morning. Lily and I went over to Mrs. Boggs's this evening. We got some beautiful flowers.

There were 116 deaths from the fever yesterday. Mrs. B. P. Anderson has it. I am so sorry. I am reading "Ancient History" aloud to Mama every day.

September 6, 1878

Papa is sick. Whether he has yellow fever or not, I don't know. Mr. Boggs came here and is going to send the doctor out, but he hasn't come yet. We went down to Mr. B's this morning to get some sage to make some tea. The doctor came just at night. Papa had the fever unmistakably and we were all likely to have it. Oh! I do hope and pray we won't any more of us have it. Papa is getting along very comfortably.

September 7, 1878

Mama fainted last night—was sick afterwards and had to go to bed. Miss McKain and Susie sat up all night. Papa is still comfortable. The doctor said he would have a light case. Mr. and Mrs. Baskin went away yesterday. Mr. Boggs was here this morning. He is so good. There were 100 new cases and 100 deaths yesterday. The doctor came today about 12 o'clock and said Papa was getting along splendidly, but tonight he is not so well. Oh! I am so sorry.

September 8, 1878

Papa is not so well. He didn't sleep a bit last night and cannot get to sleep now. Mrs. Anderson died at Hernando yesterday of yellow fever. Oh! How I feel for poor Katie. There were 137 new cases and 97 deaths yesterday. The doctor came and said Papa was getting along very well. I am so glad. His fever ought to leave him tonight. Haven't any more of us got it yet. I do hope we won't have it.

The temperature soared into the nineties during the first week of September, as Memphis sank even deeper into the morass. The city government and board of health ceased to exist; those public officials who had not succumbed to the fever fled into the countryside. Notably, the mayor and chief of police remained at their posts, though they had fewer and fewer levers of influence to affect the epidemic. Soon they, too, were dead.

Black clouds constantly hung over the city, the result of the booming cannons that had been imported from Arkansas to battle the disease. Many felt that the huge cannon balls would purify the atmosphere as they arched skyward and then fell into the river. Also contributing to the pollution were hundreds, perhaps thousands, of barrels of burning tar that were maintained by citizens in the hope they would help purify the air.

One of the biggest problems was disposing of the bodies. Coffins containing corpses were stacked on city streets to await transport to burial. One Sunday a group of grief-stricken survivors, with flowers in hand, went to Elmwood Cemetery to visit the fresh graves of their loved ones, only to discover that the graves could not be found. The sad truth was that their loved ones lay among the hundreds of coffins that were stacked at the cemetery to await burial. With so many to bury—and so few grave diggers to carry out the task—coffins were left for days at a time in the hot sun. Often, despite the availability of private graves that had been paid for in advance, the coffins were dumped into long, narrow ditches, which were then quickly covered with dirt. On any given day, heartbroken men and women could be seen wandering about the cemetery, many with flowers to place on the graves of their loved ones, only to discover that their loved ones had been relegated to an eternity of anonymity.

The *Washington Post* interviewed a physician who had just returned to Washington from Memphis, where he had helped treat the sick. He told the newspaper that there was such a shortage of nurses that white women were forced to take black men as caregivers, a situation that had resulted in sexual activity between whites and blacks. Outraged that such a thing would be printed about the city, the *Memphis Appeal* responded with an editorial that challenged the story: "No man, white or black, would be allowed to breathe after such crime became known; no such crime has been committed; white women have not been reduced to the necessity of taking Negro men for nurses; the statement is a libel upon the Negroes of Memphis, all honor to them; they have done their duty; they have acted by us nobly as policemen, as soldiers, as well as nurses; they have responded to every call made upon them in proportion to their numbers quite as promptly as the whites. A few of them threatened trouble about food at one time, but they were at the moment suppressed by a company of citizen soldiers of their own color. The colored people of Memphis, as a body, deserve well of their white fellow-citizens; we appreciate, and are proud of them." That was a position that received considerable support in the city, as evidenced by an unidentified letter writer who noted: "As far as the blacks are concerned, they have nobly fought for their rations. But this must be said: they have behaved with a quiet patience characteristic of the race, deserving all praise. All the private residences, with all their valuable contents, of Memphis, from the beginning of the great plague have been in the sole charge of the blacks. Their fidelity to their trusts will never be forgotten. No race of people on earth were ever truer."

Along with the physicians and nurses, the African Americans, and the elected officials who refused to desert their posts, the group that never faltered was the Memphis religious community, which paid a heavy price for its devotion to duty. Catholic priests and nuns, Protestant ministers, and Jewish rabbis all died in staggering numbers as they administered to the spiritual and health needs of their congregations.

At noon, one of eight Sisters of Saint Mary, all members of the Protestant Episcopal Sisterhood who had traveled to Memphis, returned to the residence and found Sister Constance resting on a sofa in the parlor. "I knew at once that she was very ill," she later wrote.[15] "She insisted that it was only a slight headache, and would not listen to my entreaties that she would go to bed, but continued dictating letters to Mrs. Bullock [an associate], who sat writing at her side. Her face was flushed with the fever; she allowed me to get a pillow and make her somewhat more comfortable, but she talked of resuming her work among the sick as soon as possible.

"I called in Dr. Armstrong as he passed the house. 'I have not the fever,' she said to him, 'it is only a bad headache; it will go off at sunset.' When told that she must go to bed, she called Mrs. Bullock to her assistance, to spare the Sisters." The sisters attempted to move her to a comfortable mattress, but she refused, saying, "It is the only one you have in the house, and if I have the fever you will have to burn it."

"It seemed as if she would keep her pledge of poverty to the last," the sister continued. "Within the same hour in which we put her to bed, Sister Theckla came in from the death bed of a poor woman. She said at once, calmly and quietly 'I am so sorry, Sister, but I have the fever. Give me a cup of tea, and then I shall go to bed.' Like Sister Constance, and for the same reason, she refused to have the mattress; the same practical spirit animated these two brave, thoughtful women.

"I was obliged to tell each Sister that the other was ill, as each wanted the other to come to her. When Dr. Armstrong came in, at eight o'clock, he pronounced both sisters ill with the fever. At nine o'clock that evening Flora Grey, the only other member of our household, was taken with the fever; her mother had died that morning. The next morning, both Sisters were very ill, their fever very high, Sister Constance unconscious most of the time. She said to me once, 'I shall never get up from my bed.'" The following day, Dr. Armstrong told the sisters that there was no hope for either Sister Constance or Sister Theckla. Within hours, the doctor's prediction came true—both sisters, along with a third one, died.

Also hard hit were the newspapers. Herbert Landrum, one of

two editors at the *Avalanche*, died on September 11 at the home of his parents. "Like his father, the reverend pastor of the Central Baptist Church, he knew no fear where duty was to be performed," wrote Louisville physician J. P. Dromgoole. "He stood his post and braved all the terrors of the epidemic, not only performing his own accustomed labors, but taking on cheerfully the load that others dropped as they died or fled from the plague."[16] Landrum's coeditor, R. A. Thompson, died a week earlier, shortly before he was to take over as Memphis postmaster. There were so many deaths at the *Memphis Appeal* that longtime editor J. M. Keating was forced to publish the newspaper with the help of only one employee, a printer.

Sensing a void in news coverage, several newspapers sent reporters to the city so there would not be a lapse in news coverage for the rest of the country. Among those present was a reporter for the *Chicago Tribune*, who dispatched these observations after roaming the streets of the nearly deserted city:

> As I write this evening the air is filled with poisonous gases from the body of a negress, "Jenny," who was employed as a cook at a boarding house at the corner of Third and Madison Streets. Her remains are supposed to have lain where they were found—in a shed, abutting on an alley to the rear of the Appeal office—for nearly ten days, as that was the last time she was seen alive. The body, bloated and eaten by rats, presented a hideously repulsive appearance, and the sickening stench is only partially dissipated by a lump of camphor in front of me. A short time back the house occupied by a respectable resident of the northern portion of the city was noticed as "smelling." Upon entering the house the wife and mother was found occupying a chair at the center of the room, with her infant child, its lips fastened in a death-grasp to the mother's nipple, dead and decomposing. The husband and father, on his back in the bed, had been dead for some time with the vomit glued to the wall in black masses, as it came from his stomach. The son lay dead on the floor.[17]

Charley Silvers, a section boss on the Mississippi and Tennessee Railway, was on his way into the city when he discovered a nude woman on a bridge, her body bleeding from briar and thorn scratches. After talking to her, he decided that she was quite insane. He found some clothing for her and took her to one of the refugee camps just outside the city, where she was questioned further.

There, camp officials learned that she was the wife of an engineer with the Mississippi and Tennessee Railway who had died of the fever two weeks earlier; they withheld that information, fearful it would worsen her already fragile emotional state. As it turned out, she already knew about her husband's death. When told two weeks earlier, she had suffered a nervous breakdown, descending into an emotional state so frightening to her friends that they kept her confined to her room. One night she escaped through a window and was not discovered missing for a long time. Disoriented, she set out to find one of the refugee camps, convinced that her husband was there, alive. Along the way, she discarded her clothing, walking nude along the railway tracks until she was discovered by Silvers. Once camp officials knew her identity, they contacted her friends and made arrangements for them to take her home.

In the midst of the chaos, Belle Wade continued to exist in what must have been a parallel universe. She left the house frequently, but she never seemed to venture far:

September 9, 1878

Papa is better this morning and his fever is leaving him. A woman died across the street from here this morning of Yellow Fever. All the Dry Goods stores are shut up and all the grocery stores on Main Street but one. The Dr. says Papa's fever had left him and he is getting along nicely. It rained nearly all the evening.

September 10, 1878

Papa is getting along very well. Feel dreadful this morning. Mama is afraid I have got the Fever and wants me to go to bed, but I am not going until I am obliged to. Do hope I have not got it. It has been raining ever since I got up.

September 12, 1878

When the Dr. came Tuesday he said I had fever and must go to bed. I hated it, but as he said so, I had to. I was real sick all the rest of the day and yesterday, but today I felt so much better when the Dr. came, I asked him couldn't I get up and he said yes if I felt well enough. I got up but I don't feel near as well as I did before I got up. Susie was taken sick yesterday, but she hasn't any fever. Papa is getting on very nicely. The doctor says he can [get] up in five days. It cleared off yesterday and has turned very cold.

September 13, 1878

Papa is getting on nicely. Susie is up and I feel very well. It is still real cold almost like winter. I never did know it to be so cold this time of year before. There were ninety-eight deaths yesterday.

*   *   *

With the arrival of October came new hope. Memphians knew little about the causes of yellow fever or its proper treatment. All they knew was that history had taught them that the disease always made a hasty exit with the arrival of the first frost, knowledge that kept everyone referring to their *Farmer's Almanac* on a regular basis to determine the most likely date of the first visible sign of the arrival of winter.

Even without a frost, there was word that help was on its way. On September 10, the citizens of Washington, DC, organized the Yellow Fever National Relief Commission, a charitable organization through which they hoped to distribute food, clothing, and money to those in need. The commission asked the War Department for the use of a ship to carry provisions on a journey from Cairo, Illinois, to New Orleans, where virtually all river and sea-going traffic had been suspended, with a stopover in Memphis. The War Department refused to supply the group with a ship, but it did approve the use of two army lieutenants, Hiram Benner and Charles Hall, who had volunteered to lead the expedition.

Once the commission made its agenda known to the public, contributions flooded in from Baltimore, San Francisco, Chicago, New York, Philadelphia, Milwaukee, and other cities. Twenty thousand dollars in cash was raised, along with 288 cases of Budweiser beer, 121 gallons of whiskey, and 1,500 quarts of champagne. The *John M. Chambers*, a paddle wheeler based in St. Louis, was charted to carry four hundred tons of ice, food, and supplies. On October 4, the ship, flying a yellow flag bearing the words "National Relief Boat," headed downriver to Memphis under the command of Lieutenant Benner, reaching its destination on October 7, where it was greeted with great enthusiasm.[18] Unfortunately, Benner became ill shortly after leaving Memphis and died of yellow fever during a stopover in Vicksburg. Upon receiving that news, the War Department ordered the ship to return to its port of origin.

Meanwhile, the epidemic raged on in Memphis, still claiming the lives of one hundred or more persons each day. Despite the stopover of the *Chambers*, fresh food supplies were rapidly being exhausted. Dr. Michael Keating, a New York physician who had traveled to Memphis to treat the sick, came down with yellow fever in October. At first, the nurses and physicians thought it was a light case, but Keating was so exhausted from the long hours he had put in with his patients that the disease quickly escalated to the black-vomit stage. "He proved himself not only the most conscientious of physicians, but the best of friends," wrote Dr. J. P. Dromgoole. "[But] he yielded rapidly, and he sank quietly but consciously into the sleep that knows no waking. His mind which had been a little clouded early on Thursday morning, was clear at the last, and the keenness of penetration which served him to predict with accuracy as he did, the hour at which his eyes would close upon the world. . . . Our call for physicians reached him while pursuing the even tenor of his way in modest practice. He could not resist so urgent an appeal from the people he loved so well, and he ventured all he had of prospect and of life, and died on the doctors' battle field, crowned with the double honors of hero and of martyr."[19]

Louis Daltroff, a Howard Association undertaker, worked at night at the cemetery, digging graves and burying the dead. He tried to ignore the rain that pelted him hour after hour, hoping to get home to a warm bed at a decent hour. At midnight, he was handed a telegram from someone connected with the house of Menkin & Brother. The message asked him to pick up the body of a young employee, a Jew, and then bury him in the Jewish cemetery. Daltroff made a midnight run to the hospital, where bodies were piled on each other, mattresses and all, as they died. It took more than an hour for him to move the bodies, all in the last stages of putrefaction, and locate the one he sought. Although the city was deserted at that time of night, he loaded the body into his wagon and drove it to the Jewish cemetery, where he dug the grave himself. That same morning, at four o'clock, he was back at work at his original cemetery, digging graves.

Among those coming down with the fever was Belle Wade, who neglected her diary during her illness, but then returned to it with renewed enthusiasm on October 12:

> I have been sick with the fever for twelve days. I had a very light case. My fever lasted only forty-eight hours, but I had to stay in bed. I got up the tenth day, dressed and went in the next room— stayed about ten minutes and fainted, so of course I had to go back to bed. I sat up a good while yesterday and I wrote a letter to Willie from whom I got a letter the day before. I have been up

nearly all day today. I was taken [ill] Tuesday, the 1st and dear little Henry [Belle's younger brother] was taken the 4th. Oh! He has been so sick. His fever was very high indeed and after that left him, he had black vomit, but through the blessing of God and good nursing he is now better—though not out of danger. The dear little darling was at the point of death for several days. The doctors didn't think he could possibly get well, but I am so thankful he is better now.

We had two nurses for him—a man and a woman. The latter is a splendid nurse and thinks a great deal of Henry which is a good thing. We had two doctors for him, too—Dr. Alex Erskine and Dr. McFarland of Savannah, Georgia. Poor Lily was taken last Sunday. She has been very ill, also. There was one night they thought she would die, but she, too, is better now, though not out of danger. I feel so thankful that I had a mild case, that I can hardly express my gratitude to God for being so merciful to me. Dear Papa had got over his fever, but has had to sit up so much lately and has had so much anxiety that he [is] not so well as he would have been. He says he thinks he will go up town Monday if nothing happens. Miss McKain is alright again. I am glad of that.

Belle Wade had only two more entries in her diary. On October 13, she wrote: "I stayed up all day today and felt very well. Henry is getting on only tolerably well—poor dear little fellow—how he has suffered. Dear Papa had a chill last night, but is feeling better today. Lily is getting on very well." Belle's final entry appeared on October 14: "I stayed up all day again today and went outdoors. I am so thankful I am able to go out. Henry was worse last night. His pulse went down so low Mama thought he would surely die, but he is better this morning. Papa went up town today for the first time. He said he felt very well when he came home."

Belle, along with her 136-page diary with its poignant and chilling view of an epidemic that brought pain and suffering to so many thousands, survived the ordeal, but it seems odd that she did not record in her diary the jubilation associated with the disease's exit. Perhaps she was simply too exhausted to give it any more thought.

On October 16, two days after Belle Wade's last entry, Jefferson Davis Jr., son of the former president of the Confederacy, died of yellow fever at five o'clock in the evening. Like so many others, Jefferson Davis and his wife had fled to the Mississippi countryside to escape the epidemic; their only son, affectionately referred to as Jeff Davis, was in Louisville, Kentucky, with his married sister. When she let it be known that she was returning to be with her husband, who had remained in Memphis, Jeff offered to accompany her. When word first reached Jefferson Davis of his son's illness, both he and his wife prepared to return to Memphis, only to be discouraged by a close friend who offered to go to the city to look after Jeff. Unfortunately, he arrived too late. Jefferson Davis Jr. was laid to rest the following day in Elmwood Cemetery with a funeral that was attended by fifteen to twenty people, said to be the largest gathering for a burial since the epidemic began. With the death of Jeff Davis went the former president's last hope of seeing his name perpetuated in the next generation, marking the end of an old way of life.

*   *   *

The frost that Memphis had eagerly awaited occurred on October 19. The following day, the *Memphis Appeal,* which had never missed a single issue despite the loss of all employees except the editor and a printer, announced the end of the yellow fever epidemic. An editorial proclaimed: "The epidemic is over. The Board of Health officially declares so, and invites absentees to return. Business will doubtless be fully resumed by the end of the week and by November we will, we have reason to hope, be on the full tide of prosperity again."

In its enthusiasm, the newspaper jumped the gun, but under the circumstances its optimism is understandable. With that first killing frost, the number of yellow fever cases dropped dramatically so that by October 28 authorities were comfortable declaring an official end to the epidemic. Of the nearly twenty thousand residents who remained in Memphis during the epidemic, seventeen thousand contracted the disease—with 5,150 confirmed deaths, most of which occurred among white residents. Of the fourteen thousand African Americans who remained in the city, less than one thousand died. Of the 111 physicians in the city when the epidemic began, fifty-four came down with the disease, and thirty-three died.

Within days of the announcement, the refugee camps were disbanded, businesses reopened their doors, the Memphis & Louisville railroad put its trains on a double schedule to accommodate all the people returning from the north, and the port was again filled with barges awaiting cotton shipments. Watching the activity at the wharf, a reporter for the Memphis *Avalanche* remarked: "To look at the immense piles of freight of every description, no one could imagine the desolation and dread silence that reigned supreme where now is heard the noise of hundreds of wagons and drays." It was a sight that brought joy to the hearts of the directors of the cotton exchange, who met on November 5 for the first time since August.

When the final cost of the epidemic was calculated, it was placed at $15 million. A more long-range effect, of course, was the manner in which the epidemic tilted the racial politics of the city. Not only did African Americans have a greater survivoral rate during the epidemic, they emerged with a destiny that would eventually provide them with an even greater challenge—control of the city's political and social future.

*   *   *

Memphis residents had only a brief time to bask in their deliverance from the scourge of yellow fever. The learned in December that the city's tax base had been cut in half, with many citizens unable to pay their taxes. Memphis was bankrupt.

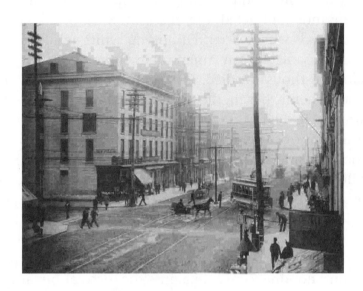

Memphis's Main Street at the turn of the century.

In January 1879, the state of Tennessee revoked Memphis's charter, which meant that it ceased to exist as a city. Instead, it was declared a taxing district under the control of state officials. Residents were provided with fire and police protection, health and sanitation protection, and public works. Furthermore, the city was placed on an austere budget until it was able to satisfy its creditors.

The winter and spring months were bleak for most Memphians as the realization set in that they had lost thousands of citizens, many of them respected leaders in the community, and they had lost financial standing in the marketplace. There was no money with which to rebuild and no credit with which to borrow money. Serious consideration was given to simply abandoning the city and starting over in a new location.

Throughout the spring and early summer of 1879, there were rumors that yellow fever had returned to the city. The *Avalanche* attributed the rumors to "crack-brained persons." A sense of unease fell over the city as the survivors of 1878 examined every illness and complaint in their neighborhoods as possible danger signs. Then, on July 9, the unthinkable happened—Frank Mulbrandon, a shoemaker, died under suspicious circumstances, and his death was confirmed to be the result of yellow fever. Word spread quickly, and by the following day all roads and trains were jammed with people fleeing the city. Dire bulletins raced over telegraph wires, causing cities such as New Orleans; Galveston, Texas; and Cairo, Illinois, to quarantine Memphis.

Reacting to that news, the *Washington Post* observed: "There is reason to fear the development of yellow fever at Memphis is but the dirge-like prelude to another appalling tragedy in that most unfortunate of American communities."

The Tennessee Health Board declared that the city was again in an epidemic, and citizens were advised to leave the city and not return until further notice. Steps were taken to locate and then isolate new victims of the fever. Flags were placed in front of homes in which the disease was suspected, and no one was allowed to leave or enter the homes, except with the approval of the board. When a call went out for help from other communities, the same Memphis newspapers that had played such an important role in the city's survival the previous year seemed to snap under the pressure. The *Avalanche* wrote: "Beggars all. Shall we be beggars all? God forbid." This time around, the atmosphere was poisoned with words, not burning tar and cannon shot. The Howards barred the press from its meetings in an effort to stem the bad publicity.

Still, the news trickled out to the public, this story with a Nashville dateline: "Yesterday 51 little orphans arrived here from the St. Mary's home in Memphis in charge of one of the sisters. All the little ones been thrown onto the charity of the world, having lost any relatives who could rear them in the yellow fever epidemic. A crowd gathered at the depot to welcome them. . . . All were given new clothes and those which they wore up here were burned."[20]

Those kinds of stories irritated Memphians to no end. They were happy that fifty-one orphans were able to be cared for, but it galled them to no end that their biggest competitor for state influence, Nashville, would seem to gloat over Memphis's inability to provide homes for its needy children.

The state health board, which was based in Nashville, further inflamed passions by establishing a picket guard around the city. Called "Rule No. 6," the board's order mandated that "neither lint cotton nor seed cotton will be allowed to enter Memphis during the epidemic." Businesses and citizens dependent on the cotton trade reacted bitterly, but the board refused to rescind its order. Halfway through September, Memphis resembled a Civil War city under siege. Public gatherings, even church services, were prohibited, which meant that members of the Howard Society, physicians and nurses, grave diggers, newspaper reporters, and armed militia officers were just about the only people allowed to be on the streets.

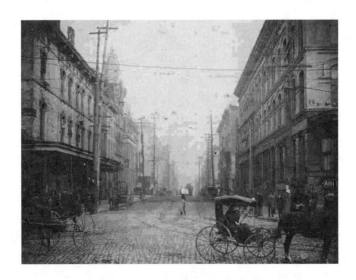

Downtown Memphis at the turn of the century.

Memphis was isolated from the rest of the world, with strict orders that no one could enter or leave the city, a situation that kept the newspapers near the boiling point. Wrote the *Avalanche*: "Memphis has been literally destroyed by . . . the National [Health Board] and the State Board. If the remorseless tyranny of these two organizations is to be continued indefinitely, it will be a wise proceeding to burn the town."

By the time the first frost arrived, it was apparent that the 1879 epidemic had been far less severe than the one that had crippled the city the previous year, totaling fewer than two thousand cases and only 595 lives. However, because it lasted longer than the 1878 epidemic—and resulted in the stunting of an already crippled economy—it may have been more disastrous than its predecessor.

Despite its handicaps, Memphis fought back, using cotton as the building block for its uncertain future. From a population of 33,592 in 1880, it bounded to 102,320 by 1900. Although the yellow fever epidemics of 1878 and 1879 destroyed the city's ambition to become the premier city in the South, it did set the stage for what may end up being its most enduring legacy, the discovery of W. C. Handy's blues. On record as having experienced the most devastating urban disaster in American history, what better city to be named the "Birthplace of the Blues"?

CHAPTER FOUR

mississippi devastated by yellow jack

There isn't much that Natchez, Mississippi, hasn't seen in its long history. First visited by Spanish conquistador Hernando de Soto, who died just north of the city in 1542, it was later visited by French explorer Robert de LaSalle, who went on to discover what would one day be known as New Orleans. Of course, Natchez already had existed for hundreds of years as a village inhabited by the Natchez Indians.

When the French established the first white settlement there in 1714, its uniqueness extended not just to its geographical trademark—a two-hundred-foot bluff that overlooked the Mississippi River—but to its distinction as the only white settlement on the entire length of the river. The Natchez Indians were quickly pushed away from the river to make room for hundreds of African slaves and their owners, planters who had visions of creating the largest plantations in the world.

Natchez was governed by the French until it was ceded to the British in the Treaty of Paris (1763). The settlement remained under British control until it was surrendered to Spain in 1799, when the settlement was admitted to the American union. It was populated mainly by Scottish, Irish, and British loyalists who went west to escape the colonies because they still felt an allegiance to the British monarchy and had a kinship with the planters over the slave issue. Individual rights were not popular with these settlers because they argued that some men, by virtue of their wealth and social standing, were more equal than others. By the time Mississippi became a territory, Natchez was home to an assortment of riverboat captains and sailors, Indians, explorers, and wealthy plantation owners who felt great antipathy toward America's "liberal" agenda, military officers, and storekeepers, of all of Natchez's inhabitants took great delight in their status as rebels who lived on the far side of civilization.

At first glance, Mississippi's first territorial governor, Winthrop Sargent, a Massachusetts-born graduate of Harvard University who had served in the Continental Army, seemed to run counter to the popular will of the people under his jurisdiction, but he was not in his new post long before it became evident that one of his guiding principles was a deeply held belief that the races should remain segregated. Since there were few, if any, free blacks in Natchez—and social integration was not an issue among slaves—his segregationist efforts were directed toward the Indians.

The Natchez Indians already had been pushed away from the bluffs into the bush, but they were a small tribe compared with the mighty Choctaw, who, along with the Chickasaw in northern Mississippi, owned most of the land. Sargent sought to control the Choctaw by reducing the number of Indians that would be permitted to enter the city.

"It will be well, I think, to be very sparing of passports for Indians to visit white people, and to confine them to chiefs and men of real consequence amongst the tribes, for the less we mix, the better the prospect of harmony," Sargent wrote. "Horse stealing, robberies, and murders, may in some measure thereby be avoided, and our friendship of course, longer continued."[1]

Not surprisingly, the proud Choctaw took exception to Sargent's segregationist policy. They had intermarried with whites for decades without protest from white leaders, and they saw no reason to change their behavior. Neither did working-class whites and slaves. Despite government policy, Indians, slaves, and whites mingled and conducted business as usual, a fact of life that soon enough became apparent to Sargent, who then became obsessed with forming a militia to protect the Mississippi territory. He declared a military draft that required all free men between the ages of sixteen and fifty to be inducted into service. They received no training, but they were required to parade through the city on the first Saturday of each month, pausing only long enough to fire their rifles and make a few jabs at imaginary targets with their bayonets.

Sargent's obsession with security was based on a belief that racial intermingling among the tens of thousands of Indians and slaves would lead to a revolt. As an outsider to the region, he assumed, incorrectly, that all conflict was based on race. He understood neither the Indians nor the black slaves. In truth, neither group was likely to stage a revolt against the white settlers.

For years, the Shawnee chiefs had tried to persuade the Choctaw to join them in a war against the Americans, but Choctaw Chief Pushmataha, who believed that his people could live in peace with the whites, refused to form an alliance with the Shawnee. He was especially grateful to the Americans for assisting the Choctaw during an epidemic, believed to be yellow fever. Chief Pushmataha explained it this way: "These white Americans buy our skins, our corn, our cotton, our surplus game, our baskets and other wares. . . . They have encouraged and helped us in the production of our crops. They have taken many of our wives into their homes to teach them useful things. They pay for their work, while learning. . . . They doctored our sick. They clothed our suffering. They fed our hungry."

By 1808 Natchez was considered the most remote corner of the American frontier. We would know little about the city itself if it were not for an American investor named Christian Schultz, who set out from New York in 1807 to explore the potential of the

Ohio wilderness. He traveled to Natchez by way of the Ohio River, which begins where the Allegheny and Monongahela rivers meet in the city of Pittsburgh, and then empties into the Mississippi River at what is now Cairo, Illinois.

Schultz's observations of Natchez in 1808 are revealing:

> From the best information I could obtain, this city contains nearly three hundred houses, and about three thousand inhabitants, including all colors. There are several extensive mercantile houses established here, and one at least which imports goods directly from England. There are two printing offices, and consequently two newspapers, which are published weekly. The buildings in general are neat, yet I found none within the town that can be considered elegant. The principal hotels are upon a genteel establishment, yet not in a style corresponding to the general character of the place for luxury: but to a Mississippi sailor, who like an alligator may be said to have lived in mud while upon the river, they afford no trifling luxury. The streets of Natchez are not paved, nor have they even the convenience of a paved sidewalk; consequently in wet weather it must be disagreeable walking. As the city, however, is situated on the summit of the hills . . . the water from rain passes off very readily, and a bright sun in a few hours absorbs the remaining moisture.[2]

Governor Sargent came under frequent attack for his rigid views on separating the races and for his determination to militarize the population. The people who had settled there had their own ways of doing things, and Sargent's attempts to change came under stiff opposition. When Thomas Jefferson defeated President John Adams in the presidential election, Sargent traveled to Washington in 1801 to argue for his reappointment as governor. Jefferson heard him out and then fired him, appointing William Clairborne as his replacement. Clairborne was well known to Jefferson, first as a patriot whose entire family had supported the Revolution and second as his personal clerk. Jefferson was not casual in his appointment; he invariably chose individuals he knew and trusted. Clairborne proved to be quite popular among local residents. He was a handsome man who wore his close-cropped hair in the style made famous by Napoleon. He backed away from Sargent's rigid social engineering, but he showed equal paranoia when it came to maintaining a militia, and he was equally unrelenting with the Indians.

In one of his most famous confrontations with the Choctaw, he gathered the leaders at a government house in Natchez to lecture them on their perceived moral shortcomings. "It is my way to speak straight," he said. "Listen then to what I say, and hold fast my talk. The white people have made to me of late, many complaints. . . . Brothers, I hope none of you are guilty of these acts. . . . I am going to give you some good advice. Quit drinking whiskey, for it will make you fools and old women. Return to your own land and make bread for your families . . . while you remain in our settlements, you shall not have one ounce of flour from me."

Two years into Clairborne's appointment, he was asked by President Jefferson to travel to New Orleans to receive the Louisiana Purchase from France. He was appointed governor of the Territory of Orleans, where he served until Louisiana was admitted into the union, at which point he was elected the state's first governor. After he left Natchez, Mississippi became the union's twentieth state in 1817, with Natchez chosen as the capital. (Subsequently, the capital was moved to Washington and then to Jackson.) The first census, taken in 1817, identified twenty-three thousand slaves, twenty-five thousand whites, and thirty-five thousand Native Americans in Mississippi.

Clairborne had several low-level successes as governor—the founding of a college that he named after Jefferson and a survey of the Natchez and Mobile districts—but his most enduring accomplishment was the establishment of a mail route on the Natchez Trace, a two-thousand-year-old wilderness trail that stretches five hundred miles, from Natchez to Nashville. The

French mapped the existing trail in the early 1700s, but it was created by Native Americans long before the discovery of America. There are existing mounds on the trace that date to 100 BCE.

In 1810 the trace was the most heavily traveled wilderness trail in the Southwest. Clairborne's designation of the trace as a mail route provided it with a legitimacy it lacked as a mere Indian trail and gave travelers who used it as an overland route from Washington to New Orleans the comfort of knowing that the road was protected by the United States Government. Today, it is a federal park.

There was a downside, however. The Indians initially made the path next to rivers, lakes, and ponds so that travelers would have easy access to water. As a result, portions of the trace cut through swampy areas that harbor thick swarms of insects such as mosquitoes. During the yellow fever epidemics in New Orleans, it was common for those fleeing the city to travel to Natchez so that they could then travel by foot to Nashville and beyond. Not surprisingly, yellow fever cases sprang up all along the trace, transporting the disease into the Mississippi heartland.

No one knows for sure when yellow fever first appeared in Natchez and the surrounding territory. Indian records make it clear that plagues were a regular occurrence among the Natchez and Choctaw, though it is unknown whether the illnesses were yellow fever, cholera, or an assortment of other fever-related diseases.

Natchez was boxed in by the disease long before actual cases appeared. In 1765 there was a documented epidemic in Pensacola, Florida, of real concern because Pensacola was not far from the coastal boundary of what later became the Mississippi Territory. The epidemic, which appeared shortly after a British garrison took possession of the province of Florida, was traced to British soldiers who arrived in the port from England by way of the West Indies.

With the first recorded yellow fever epidemic in New Orleans occurring in 1796—and returning in 1812, 1817, and 1818 before making a major statement in 1819—there were certainly fears of an epidemic in Natchez throughout the early 1800s. A wealthy planter created a controversy in 1818 when he raised questions about Natchez's status as a safe refuge from yellow fever. A spirited public debate ensued in the local newspapers, ending with the conclusion that the city was safe because of its distance from New Orleans (about 350 miles).

One of the first serious epidemics in Mississippi took place in Woodville, the site of Jefferson Davis's Rosemont Plantation, which had been established in 1810 near the coast, not far from the boundary that separated Mississippi and Louisiana. Early in July 1844, a Mr. Thurber left Galveston, Texas, and traveled to Woodville by way of New Orleans, arriving in the Mississippi community (population nine hundred) on July 12. Upon his arrival, he took lodgings with Colonel J. S. Lewis in a large brick building with a well-shaded yard that was located near the railroad depot. He took rooms upstairs in the front part of the house, where there were large windows that opened onto the front yard.

On the day after his arrival, Thurber became ill before going to bed. Once it was known that he had yellow fever, the doctors in town became interested in who visited the Lewis home after Thurber's arrival, for it was their firm belief that the disease was passed from person to person, whether by direct contact or by breathing the same air. Dr. Andrew Kilpatrick, a local physician who treated the second yellow fever case in town, later wrote an article for the *New Orleans Medical Journal* about the epidemic. Titled "An Account of the Yellow Fever Which Prevailed in Woodville, Mississippi in the Year 1844," it reads like a Sherlock Holmes mystery and goes into great detail about the physician's thought process in solving the mystery. One of the first things he did, as the number of cases quickly escalated, was to trace the whereabouts of every patient in relation to Colonel Lewis's house.

Regarding the visit of the second yellow fever patient, a Mr.

Collins, to the Lewis home, Dr. Kilpatrick wrote: "It might be asked though, by some, how could the halitus [sic] from Mr. Thurber's room, above stairs, affect the air in the porch? Mr. Collins' visit was late in the afternoon, when the moisture and density of the atmosphere might very well favor the transit of the miasma; and besides, Colonel Lewis had been in his room to attend to the wants of the sick man, and the halitus might easily be carried about, for so short a distance, in the clothes of Lewis, and other members of his family, and diffused into the air around. However, the case of Mr. Collins does not materially affect the merits of the question, as it is admitted on all hands, that Mr. Thurber was the first case in town, and it is demonstrable, by the list of cases furnished by Dr. Stone, that it spread from him, and attacked those who visited the family."[3]

Dr. Kilpatrick then goes on to take exception to Dr. Stone's assessment of the epidemic. "In the list furnished by Dr. Stone he seems to wish to fix each individual to one spot, so any yards away from Thurber, and to forget that in a place, the size of this, where nearly everybody is acquainted if not familiar, there must of necessity be much intercourse in various ways," he wrote. "He seems to endow Mr. Thurber with an exclusive patent for yellow fever, and if a person has not visited him, that they could not possibly contract it elsewhere."

A portion of Dr. Kilpatrick's yellow fever article also discussed the treatment he favored for the disease during the epidemic. The important treatment tool, he maintained, was venesection, or bleeding. "Few cases recovered where it had been neglected, and for success to attend its employment, it was necessary to resort to it early—the first twenty-four hours was the time specified," he wrote. "In cases of most intense agony and suffering, pulse bounding and throbbing, heart laboring like a curbed steed, and the patient rolling and tossing from side to side, and it seemed that to relieve him required superhuman skill and power, by the touch of the lancet all pain was relieved and calmed as it were by magic, and the fever would shortly vanish, never again to return."

Dr. Kilpatrick's investigation of the Woodville epidemic proved to be a fascinating letter to nowhere, for it did not bring medical knowledge any closer to solving the mystery. Ironically, he came close to understanding the disease without realizing it. Prior to discussing his investigation, he devoted space in his article to describing Woodville and the surrounding area: "Rains were very constant during the spring and summer, so much so, as to prove very irksome to our planters in the cultivation of their crops," he wrote. "The streams were repeatedly swollen beyond their banks, carried off fences, and inundated portions of the crops, which were planted in the bottoms. . . . There were vast swarms of flies early in the summer, and mosquitoes by thousands, which annoyed us incessantly. The latter were nearly as troublesome in the day as in the night, and fumigations could not expel them from the houses."[4]

Ten years after the 1844 epidemic, yellow fever again returned to Woodville. Typical of the anguish were letters written in 1855 by Susan Keller, of Woodville, to her sister, Phoebe Richardson, about the death of Richardson's son from yellow fever. "I hardly know how to commence writing as it is always painful to me to communicate sad news," Keller wrote. "The yellow fever made its appearance here the first part of September. The doctor advised all who wished to escape having it to leave town. . . . Your son John and family, among the rest left town but poor Ephriagm would not go, but chanced to stay at John's house with those that remained. . . . He was taken last Saturday morning. Sent for Doc Holt, one of the best Docs we have. . . . He died last evening at 9 o'clock p.m. and was interred this morning in the graveyard at half past 9 o'clock near his dear uncle. My son William stayed with him as much as he could. He saw that he had men to sit up with him who could be depended on. . . . He lay in John's room on a good feather bed and fire all the time in the room. . . . I wanted to see him but the Doc will not let a yellow fever patient see any one that would excite them in the least. . . . I trust that he has gone home to Heaven, far from a world of affliction and sorrow."[5]

*   *   *

Along with statehood came an influx of white settlers, all desirous of land owned by the Choctaw and Chickasaw. The Indian Removal Law provided the settlers with the ammunition they needed to impose the 1830 Treaty of Dancing Rabbit Creek on the Choctaw, which required them to relocate to Oklahoma. Thirteen thousand Choctaw made the 550-mile journey, reducing the Indian population in Mississippi to twenty-two thousand. A similar deal with the Chickasaw, who lived in northern Mississippi, reduced the total Indian population in the state to about ten thousand, thus making whites the majority race in Mississippi.

As a result, Natchez quickly became the state's premier city. By 1830 it had more millionaires per capita than any city in the United States, with most of the wealth coming from cotton and land speculation stimulated by the removal of the Indians. White settlements spread outward from Natchez to the Gulf Coast to the south, to the east and northeast into north Mississippi by means of the Natchez Trace (by 1840 the northern half of the state would have a population of 375,000), and to the north along the Mississippi River into the delta, the swampy flatlands that were home to more snakes and mosquitoes than any other part of the state.

The Mississippi Delta stretches from Memphis to Vicksburg, fertile land that was home to a sophisticated culture of Indians twelve thousand years before the arrival of the white man and his black slaves. The Indians, who had disappeared by the 1700s, lived along the Mississippi River on mounds that were high enough to protect them from floodwaters. When the first white settlers arrived in the delta in the 1830s, they quickly discovered that they, too, would have to either live on mounds or devise a system of levees that could protect them from the floodwaters that arrived almost every year during that critical time between planting and harvesting. By 1858, a stable system of levees was constructed that allowed the entire delta to be opened up to cotton planters.

In the years preceding the Civil War, Mississippi seemed on the verge of unprecedented prosperity, thanks to a booming cotton economy that poured money into the state. In 1860 personal property in Mississippi was assessed at more than $438 million, compared with $302 million in Massachusetts and $272 million in Ohio.[6] Of course, all that wealth was in the hands of only a few people, setting the stage for a rapid downfall during and after the Civil War, which left the state's economy in shambles.

At the outbreak of the Civil War, the total white population of the eleven states of the Confederacy was 5.4 million, which compared unfavorably to the North's 21 million. In terms of white men between the ages of eighteen and thirty-five, the South had only about eight hundred thousand potential soldiers, while the North had more than three million. Those are bad odds with which to enter into war, but no one in the South cared about that, especially in Mississippi.

Mississippians have never fought one war at a time. They have always fought multiple wars: the one in which they are currently engaged—and all the previous wars that have left scars on their genetic consciousness. When the battle cry arose for support of the Confederacy, very few whites in Mississippi owned slaves— only thirty-one thousand white Mississippians out of a population of three hundred fifty-three thousand whites had a personal stake in slavery.

For the men who fought the war, slavery was never the major issue. That's because white Mississippians never believed in the concept of a "United States." They believed in the life view, perpetuated by the British, that some people, by virtue of their race, breeding, and success in life, were entitled to more rights than others. That was the cause for which Mississippi sent seventy-

eight thousand white men off to war, not slavery. White Mississippians were still upset about the outcome of the War of Independence, and they believed that, if they won the Civil War, the
clock could be rolled back to prerevolutionary days, and they
could again become British subjects. It is a plantation view that
has continued into modern times, perpetuating the belief that the
Republican Party is the portal through which the Bill of Rights
can be suspended and relations with England restored to the
"good old days" that preceded the American Revolution.

When the time came for Generals Ulysses S. Grant and
William Sherman to invade Mississippi, they stuck close to the
Natchez Trace and did most of their fighting along its route, tar-
geting Tupelo, Oxford, Holly Spring, Jackson, and Natchez, then
north to Vicksburg and south to the coast. Natchez was of no
strategic importance to the Union, but it once was bombarded by
a Union gunboat that anchored just offshore and sent a small
boat ashore to collect ice for the wounded. There probably would
never have been a bombardment if local citizens had not fired on
the smaller boat.

Annie Harper, a member of a prominent plantation family,
later wrote about the bombardment: "The immediate response to
this unwarranted piece of folly was a shell from the gunboat.
From two o'clock until six the bombardment was incessant. The
roads leading from the town were filled with a stampeding
throng. . . . One circumstance alone prevented the destruction of
life and property from being immense—very few of the shells
exploded, a few went crashing through buildings full of people,
where the carnage would have been very great had they exploded.
One little girl running up the hill leading from the landing was
killed by a piece of shell."

Vicksburg, with its impressive fortifications and its capability
to stop traffic on the river with its cannons, was the major target
of the Union army. Indeed, if Vicksburg had not existed, it is
doubtful that Union forces would ever have entered Mississippi.

An invasion was the price the state paid for its one instance of military prowess.

Vicksburg was surrounded by Union forces that bombarded the city on a daily basis from across the river in an effort to break the will of its defenders. "All night long their deadly hail of iron dropped through roofs and tore up the deserted and denuded streets," wrote one survivor.[7] "For forty days and nights without interval the women and children of Vicksburg took calmly and bravely the iron storm. It became such an ordinary occurrence that I have seen ladies walk quietly along the streets while the shells burst above them, their heads protected only by a parasol held between them and the sun."

Another view of the shelling is provided by a woman who traveled to Vicksburg to be with her soldier-husband: "Very few houses are without evidence of the bombardment, and yet the inhabitants live in their homes happy and contented, not knowing what moment the houses may be rent over their heads by the explosion of a shell. 'Ah!' I said to a friend, 'how is it possible you live here?' 'After one is accustomed to the change,' she answered, 'we do not mind it. But becoming accustomed—that is the trial.' I was reminded of the poor man in an infected district who was met by a traveler and asked, 'How do you live here?' 'Sir, we die,' was the laconic reply."[8]

By the end of the war, all of Mississippi was in ruins, politically, economically, and socially. Federal victories on the battlefield destroyed all existing institutions of stability at the city and county level, replacing them with military districts that governed with an iron hand. Of the seventy-eight thousand Mississippians who fought for the Confederacy, more than fifty-nine thousand were killed or wounded. One-fifth of the state's total revenue during the first year of peace was used to purchase artificial arms and legs for returning soldiers. Federal troops prevented Confederate veterans from voting or running for elective office, which meant that the voting pool was made up almost entirely of white men who never served in the army, former male slaves, and the Republican carpetbaggers from the North who went to Mississippi to make fortunes.

The Republicans and the freed slaves made strong showings in elections after the war. Republican Ulysses S. Grant, who had been responsible for so much destruction in the state, carried Mississippi by a margin of two to one in the first presidential election held after the war. From 1869 to 1878, the office of secretary of state in Mississippi was held exclusively by African Americans, and in 1875 Mississippi elected its first black lieutenant governor. Its first black United States senator was elected in 1869.

Those are the high points of Reconstruction. On the negative side is that the occupation army cut African Americans very little slack. The army forbade freed slaves to travel without passes from their employers, and blacks were prohibited from being on the streets at night and warned about engaging in "insubordination," a polite way of saying they would be punished if they talked back to their white employers. If they violated their work contracts, any white citizen had the authority to arrest them.

One of the great success stories of postwar Mississippi was the way that delta planters, deprived almost overnight of their entire workforce, offered freed slaves generous terms as sharecroppers. Instead of flocking to the cities, freed slaves remained in what was essentially still a wilderness area, where they traded their labor for a share of the wealth, a partnership that desperate planters were eager to accept. It would take nearly a century for the sharecropper arrangement to go bad, but, for many years, it allowed African Americans to compose two-thirds of the farmers in the state.

With so much economic and social destruction to contend with throughout the state, public healthcare ceased to be a priority, which was probably just as well since the war had claimed the lives of so many of the state's physicians. Yellow fever continued at low levels throughout the war, taking lives here and there, but, with so many larger issues of concern, the disease stopped being the subject of conversation. Reconstruction was such an emotional issue for whites and blacks that it consumed the energies of those who, in years past, would have been diligent to stand guard in the war against yellow fever.

One of the most troubling aspects of Reconstruction was the tendency of freed slaves to flee to the cities from the rural areas of the state in the hope of building a new life. Unfortunately, they found few jobs, which meant that many were forced to live in poverty in crowded conditions that set the stage for a devastating return of yellow fever.

*   *   *

In May 1878, with rumors flying that yellow fever had returned to New Orleans, Mississippi state health officials sent letters to each county and city health board reminding them of the two procedures—quarantine and disinfectant—that they should follow should an epidemic spread from New Orleans. That letter was followed at the end of July with a second letter informing local officials that there were thirty-three reported cases of yellow fever in New Orleans.

Unfortunately, the letters were ignored. As New Orleans sank deeper and deeper into the worst epidemic in its history, complacent local officials throughout Mississippi did nothing to prepare for the inevitable. In fact, the first cases of yellow fever in Mississippi had already appeared when the second letter arrived.

The towboat *John Porter*, which left New Orleans on July 19 to make its regular run upriver to the Ohio River, north of Memphis, stopped in Vicksburg on July 25 to bury two crewmen, an engineer and a fireman. The ship's captain said they had died of "sunstroke." Despite already published accounts that the towboat had been the initial source of infection in New Orleans—and public speculation that the two men had died of yellow fever—a Vicksburg man named Paul Stoltz signed on to replace the fallen fireman. He was on the towboat when it passed through Memphis and he was on board when it reached Cairo, Illinois, where he first began showing symptoms of yellow fever.

Before the *John Porter* made its way back downriver, the Vicksburg *Herald* urged a quarantine of New Orleans, but local health officials did not respond. In Jackson, approximately sixty miles east of Vicksburg, residents became increasingly paranoid, prompting one newspaper to publish a story with the headline: "Jackson Believes That Vicksburg Is Concealing Yellow Fever and Has Been Some Time." The newspaper expressed "indignation" at the way Vicksburg authorities had responded to inquiries about the disease: "The belief is current in Jackson that Vicksburg has had the yellow fever for some time but on account of local pressure it has not been announced by the physicians of that place. . . . There's one thing that's been brought out prominently in the last twenty-four hours and that is that if there is an epidemic in this city the people of Jackson do not desire to have a physician sent from Vicksburg as the state health officer. . . . The council would do well to look into the Vicksburg matter and to quarantine against that town as the thing that they have been having over there seems to be very bad. The local sentiment is in favor of such an action."[9]

On August 7, Stoltz arrived back in Vicksburg, stopping at a drugstore on his way home. When asked about the deaths on the towboat, he responded, "Why, they no more had it than I have now." More convinced by his sickly appearance than by his words, local health officials hospitalized him that same day. He died two days later of yellow fever, leading the city to announce the disease's arrival on August 10.[10]

Two weeks later, the *Herald* reported: "The shadow of great woe hangs over our devoted city. The number of suffering from the pestilence is fearful. Yesterday we saw corpses hurried to the grave without attendant, and God only knows the ghastly sights and scenes of pain transpiring in Vicksburg tonight." By then the city resembled a ghost town. Businesses were closed, and there was no street traffic, other than hearses piled high with coffins, headed for the cemeteries. Barrels of tar burned on the streets, the black smoke darkening the sky. Trains hurried through town without slowing down, with passengers holding cloths over their faces to protect them from the disease, and riverboats passed at full speed, refusing to stop at the docks.

Not afraid were the Catholic Sisters of Mercy, who took over the operation of the city hospital when the chief physician informed them that he was ill. He subsequently died of yellow fever at thirty-eight, the same age his father had died of yellow fever—and his father also had been the chief physician at the hospital. The sisters were horrified by the condition of the hospital. One sister later wrote: "The hospital building was in a miserable condition, so filthy that the sisters had to recourse to shovels and wheelbarrows to clean the lower floor, particularly the pantry."[11] Normally the hospital cared for about fifty patients at a time, but, during the epidemic, daily admissions soared to more than three hundred. Treatment consisted of medicines such as calomel, mustard baths, and sponge baths with cold water and whisky. If the patient survived that, he or she was fed a diet of milk, rice, chicken broth, and lime water for about ten days after the fever subsided. Bed rest was prescribed, with an emphasis placed on securing a room with plenty of fresh air. Vicksburg was a very crowded city, with houses built with little space between them, especially in the poorer neighborhoods, so that meant that the "fresh air" prescribed by physicians entered bedrooms by way of windows that contained no screens. Outside the windows were rain barrels filled with water, small ponds, and drainage ditches, a mosquito-friendly environment that seemed benign on the surface.

One sister compared the epidemic to the last days of Pompeii. Once, while a sister was carrying a bowl of chicken soup to a jaundiced patient, he said, "Sister, put that down a moment and come here. I want something better."

Not certain what to expect, the sister placed the soup on a table and nervously asked, "What can you have better?"

"Salvation," he replied. "There must be something in the religion which produces so much kindness." The man was baptized the next morning, an event that gave him so much joy that he lay in his hospital bed and sang uplifting songs, right up to within an hour of his death.[12]

There was great jubilation when the relief ship, the *John M. Chambers*, made its way south from St. Louis under the command of thirty-four-year-old Lieutenant Hirum Benner. Filled with supplies and medicine, the ship brought hope to Vicksburg residents who were quickly running out of both food and medicine. Benner dropped off the needed materials in Vicksburg and then continued to New Orleans. On the way back upriver, Benner came down with yellow fever a few miles south of Vicksburg. He died after a single day of illness, prompting the *Herald* to reflect: "Since the inception of the plague, there has not been such a universal expression of public feeling and sympathy. There was a general suspension of business. Every store in the city was draped with mourning. Flags were hung at half mast. Church bells tolled and the entire city turned out en-masse. The boy lay in state in General's Hall until 9 p.m. and was viewed by thousands. They came of all ranks, rich and poor, black and white to pay their last respects to the brave and humble soldier whose name and memory are now coupled with the historic city of Vicksburg as long as time lasts and deeds like this are accumulated and remembered."

From Vicksburg, the epidemic fanned out across Mississippi like a prairie fire, as people infected in the river city fled to more rural locations, many of which were located near lakes, stagnant water, and meandering rivers with backwater pockets that harbored thick swarms of insects. Many people went to the coast, where they felt the steady breezes from the Gulf of Mexico would protect them from the dreaded yellow fever "germ." That wasn't the case, of course. Coastal towns such as Pascagoula, Ocean Springs, and Biloxi quickly found themselves running a parallel course with Vicksburg and New Orleans, as refugees suddenly appeared in the community.

Since it was up to individual towns to establish their own guidelines for quarantine, standards varied greatly from one community to the next. Health officials often ran into opposition from merchants, particularly hotel owners, who wanted to maintain a high level of trade with New Orleans to the west and Mobile to the east—and they could see no reason why potentially infected persons from epidemic areas should not travel to the coast, where they would need places to live and merchandise, especially food and clothing, to sustain them during their exile from their hometowns.

At the start of the epidemic, a seventy-year-old woman from North Mississippi, Mary Buford, traveled to Ocean Springs by train and boat to resolve a property dispute. She was aware of yellow fever cases in the area but apparently unconcerned. Ocean Springs still had a very lenient quarantine policy, a clear appeal to tourists. However, shortly after Mary arrived, she received a letter from her husband, Albert, who did not like the look of things: "The first thing that you know your retreat will be cut off. But I don't know enough to advise you. . . . I am getting uneasy as to how you are to get home without contracting the disease yourself or bringing it home in your clothing or trunk or [giving] it to the rest of us." By then, Mary was aware of her predicament. In an emotional letter to Albert, she wrote: "May God stay the terrible scourge ere it reaches my precious husband. I am so torn with conflicting thoughts that I am almost crazy. If I had the means to come I might bring the fever into my own family and cause sorrow instead of joy. I am advised not to attempt to but if I had our business here so that I could leave it I think I would come unless you opposed. I am not thinking of myself, it is of you."[13] As the days went by, Mary became even more concerned about her situation. In her letters, she tried to reassure her husband that health officials were using disinfectants in a liberal manner and that she was confident that the situation was under control, but she had a more difficult time convincing herself because, as the death toll in Ocean Springs rose, so did the anxiety level of the residents. Her letters became more and more like a countdown to disaster. The bad news for her husband began with the offhand remark that she was not feeling well. She followed that up with a letter that informed him that she had taken a quinine pill and was confident she would feel better soon. One of her last letters expressed her desire to be with him again: "It looks like I am floating away from you forever, the outlook is so gloomy, so sad." There was silence from Mary, as her letters stopped arriving. Then one day Albert received a telegram from the coast notifying him that Mary had died.[14]

With the spreading epidemic came a reluctance to believe the worst. Alluding to the "situation in regard to the scare," a Jackson newspaper tried to quell panic by reporting: "Another day finds Jackson still free from even a suspicion of the yellow scourge, and the confidence of the citizens that the active efforts of the authorities will keep it out is correspondingly increased. The cool weather of the last two or three days, too has contributed in no small degree to raise the hopes of many that the spread of the disease in infected places will be curtailed."

Optimism aside, Jackson moved quickly to quarantine against the outside world. No trains were allowed to stop in the city, and newspapers were ordered to suspend publication, an obvious attempt to prevent citizens from hearing reports of yellow fever. Nonetheless, yellow fever cases began to appear on August 31, with the first death occurring that day. It was enough to start a panic. Businesses closed and residents fled to the rural areas, where they thought they would be safe.

One of the rural areas that saw its population increase dramatically was Dry Grove, a crossroads community located about twenty-two miles southwest of Jackson. It seemed the perfect place to seek refuge: it was ten miles from the nearest railroad, and it was secluded to land travel to the point of being exotically remote. There were two physicians in Dry Grove and another two physicians less than four miles away. Everyone there felt safe from the ravages of yellow fever, despite reports that several residents had become ill with malaria. The physicians there felt it was malaria because in mid-August the pond that supplied the public mill with water was drained and deepened, and the soil dragged from the pond was identified by the experts as malaria-inducing deposits that had no relation to yellow fever. That assessment changed quickly enough once the ill persons displayed black vomit and died. By then, it was too late to turn back the refugees.[15]

Hearing of the pain and suffering in Dry Grove—of the first twenty-nine cases of yellow fever reported, twenty-eight died—Thomas Dabney, owner of the Burleigh Plantation, opened the doors of his home to those who were in need. Also taken into his home was a physician sent by the Howard Association of New Orleans, along with several trained yellow fever nurses.

"All the rooms in the house, not excepting the dining room and kitchen, were turned into sleeping chambers," Dabney's daughter, Susan, later wrote. "One gentleman, a prosperous citizen of Jackson himself drove a wagon filled with provisions to our door, because he could not hire a driver to do it. Over one thousand dollars were sent by the Howard Association in different cities and by friends of the family."

At first Dabney refused to allow his daughters to get involved with nursing the sick, but later, seeing their determination, he allowed them to travel with him to Dry Grove and later to nurse patients in their home. Susan was the only member of her family to come down with yellow fever, but she survived the disease and continued to nurse those in need. As time went by, it became increasingly difficult for the healthy to live among the dying.

Wrote Susan: "It was found necessary during those days of horror to keep up our spirits, by avoiding as far as possible all reference to the pestilence and its ravages. At the table, especially, such allusions were forbidden. The list of deaths occurring the night before was not to be spoken of at breakfast. Afterwards the names of friends, who had just died, passed quietly and without comment from mouth to mouth. There was no giving way to emotions. Why should we weep? We will soon follow them. Besides, there is no time for tears. The suffering and the dying are calling us. And the dead lie unburied, wrapped in blankets just as they died, across the church pews, waiting for a tardy coffin and a shallow grave."[16]

W. K. Douglas, a relief worker from Jackson who went to Dry Grove, later wrote of entering a house and finding three of four family members lying in bed, dead: "Two professional nurses were there, but not a particle of food nor any, even the most necessary, conveniences of a sick room. . . . The last stroke of that 'insatiate archer' fell at two o'clock, and I arose and dressed for the first time and watched by the silent dead until morning. The expected help not having come, I walked out from that dwelling which I had once thought never to leave alive, in search of someone to bury the dead. I passed up the deserted street in vain. At last I saw a man on horseback, and called to him."

The man told Douglas that he would help build a coffin if he could find the lumber, but when Douglas offered to strip the ceiling from a room in the house, the man told him not to do that—he would tear down an old shed to get the lumber. That evening, the coffin arrived. Along with his assistant and a physician, Douglas led the funeral procession, carrying the deceased in a wagon that they converted into a hearse.[17]

In nearby Lake, not a single family escaped without losing at least one member. R. K. Jayne, a member of a nearby community, heard about what was happening in Lake and went to assist the dying, though he had no friends or family there. Before dying of yellow fever in Jackson, he told of the hardships that prevented recovery and reduced the community's population by one half. Calling the treatment "unbelievably crude," he told of patients who were given no water and covered with blankets and allowed to burn with fever.

In Macon, a small town east of Jackson, near Philadelphia, Julie Raine wrote a letter to her infant daughter detailing their predicament. She and the baby's father left Memphis, she explained, in the hope they would escape the epidemic. But, she realized, the epidemic had caught up with them in Macon.

"We are hemmed in on every side—there seems no escape," she wrote. "We have not the money to obtain trains to go far into the mountains and the railroad cars are as dangerous as can be. This is our position tonight, my Baby. Tomorrow we may be numbered with the many hundreds who have already departed—victims, victims of this loathsome disease."[18] Clearly convinced that both she and her husband would succumb to yellow fever, she continued:

> I cannot bear the thought darling that I should be taken away forever without leaving some message for you, something that when you are grown you can read and think of as direct from the Mother that you never knew. I want to tell you how for months before you were born, how day and night we (Papa and I) talked of your coming, wondered what you looked like and longed for the time when we should see you. Then when you were born, what a time there was! Never was such a baby. Loved and kissed and petted until you would have been utterly spoiled if you had known it. . . . I can see you now as you lie in your cradle fast asleep, unconscious, unheeding of the great storm that is lowering so darkly o'er our heads and I pray that God will always keep you just as innocent as you are now of all dark things and that living purely you will at that Last Great Day be found among God's chosen ones, an inheritor forever of the beautiful mansions above. Goodnight my darling, darling daughter—a father and mother's love and blessing are yours forever.

*   *   *

At approximately the same time that Vicksburg was exposed to its first cases of yellow fever, two women in Grenada, located about one hundred miles south of Memphis, complained of chills while walking along the street. One of the women recovered, but the other woman died seven days later after becoming jaundiced and exhibiting black vomit. The woman's physician was not alarmed. He diagnosed her aliment as congestive fever.

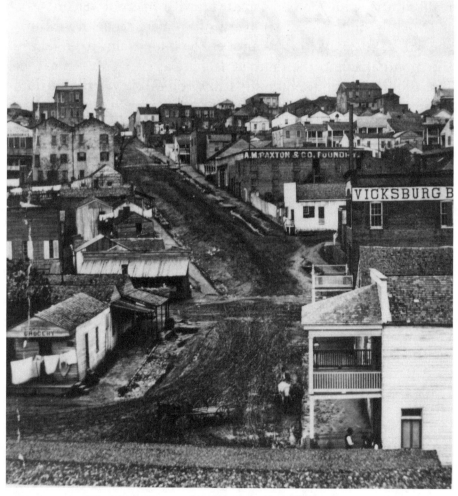

Mississippi River view of Vicksburg, Mississippi, 1876.

Less than a week later, two more fatal cases appeared—a store clerk and an inmate at the county jail. This time the deaths were diagnosed as "malignant bilious fever."[19] Several days later, a delegation of expert physicians arrived in Grenada from New Orleans and identified the mysterious illnesses as yellow fever. Once word of that fearsome diagnosis got out, the small town was overtaken by panic.

"Perhaps in the history of epidemics nothing more appalling ever occurred among civilized people than the suddenness and fatality with which it appeared in Grenada," wrote Dr. J. P. Dromgoole, the Louisville physician who went to Memphis's aid and then turned his attention to Grenada, a city of twenty-five hundred inhabitants. "Every road leading from Grenada was crowded with vehicles and horses loaded with women and children while numbers, who could not under any consideration get such conveniences, were on foot, some of them leaving mothers and fathers, sisters and brothers prostrate and dying. In many cases even the farewell was forgotten, and can never be uttered to the loved ones left behind, for in a few hours they were coffined and buried."[20]

Even as the panic spread, there were those who searched for causes of the epidemic. One woman said she was certain that it had begun with a woman whose husband had died of the plague in New Orleans; it was spread to Grenada, the woman argued, once the widow returned to the city and hung her dead husband's bedclothes out to air, thus spreading the disease. Others looked at the open ditch that ran through the center of town and emptied into the Yalobusha River. It was filled with animal carcasses, trash, and pools of stagnant water. Those who looked there for causes of the disease were close to unraveling the secret of yellow fever, but they overlooked the stagnant water in favor of the carcasses, thus their efforts to drag the animals from the ditch had no noticeable effect on the spread of the disease.

As was done in other cities, carbolic acid was used freely, and tar barrels were kept burning night and day, creating a suffocating cloud that hung over the community and crept through the alley-ways like a London fog. An item published in the *New Orleans Picayune* on August 15 painted a vivid picture: "Last night was fearful on the yellow fever victims. The death list—fourteen—was the largest since its appearance. There was great excitement during the day, many more fleeing the town. The population is now reduced to not over 300 whites. Total deaths 55: number of cases down estimated at 150. The New Orleans physicians pronounce it the most virulent type. The distress is too fearful to contemplate."[21]

As the death rate increased, people were buried in the same clothes they wore when they died. Hearses sometimes dumped remains off at the cemetery, leaving them on the ground until graves could be dug. Soon there was no food left in town. Stores closed and farmers who brought produce to town kept their wagons in barns and burned tar pots outside their houses. During his week-long visit, Dr. Dromgoole was forced to eat only bread. "The atmosphere was heavy with poison," he wrote. "It could be fairly tasted in air, and it was impossible to remove it with disinfectants."

Despite the chaos, relief supplies poured into the city—tons of ice arrived by train from Illinois, vinegar to be used as a disinfectant, paper bags that could be used by those suffering from black vomit, money to be used for coffins, and whatever food that could be shipped long distances without spoiling. As in other cities, treatment ran counter to the symptoms, often doing more harm than good. Most harmful was the practice of depriving fever patients of water. The story was told of one man who was denied water, given instead a sponge bath. Fortunately for him, his nurse was called out of the room for a moment, allowing him time to drink the dirty water in the wash pan. Another man, seeing how others begged for water, took as many jugs of water as he could carry to the top of an isolated hill and drank copious amounts of water, determined to stay there until he either died or was well enough to return home. He returned home, emaciated and weak, but very much alive.[22]

An editorial in the *Grenada Sentinel* lamented the fact that the newspaper had just enlarged its format, a proud accomplishment for a publisher, when the epidemic struck, thus obliterating, almost overnight, the newspaper's readership:

What a terrible six weeks these have been! Let fear, hope, anxiety, each and all, answer; let the dismay and flight of twelve hundred of our citizens tell; let the entire abrogation of all business speak; let the death of about two hundred and forty of our best people have its solemn voice . . . the suddenness with which it came, and the severity with which it ruled, will make it an event memorable in the history of our town and a strongly marked page in the progress of American civilization. The survivors, and we mean by that all who remained to face the appalling scourge, are coming out one by one upon the streets, like prisoners ransomed from the grave, pale, ghastly, and dispirited, yet thankful that they live to tell a tale of life and death that few have interpreted. The fearful struggle of these last six weeks, in the personal history of the sad survivors, will form an episode of anguish and terror, which the minds of those who were not present cannot realize, and the memories of those who were [here] can never forget.

When the final tally was made of the epidemic in Grenada, it revealed that nearly half the population—all but four of the people who remained in town—came down with the disease (1,050 cases reported), and of that number 350 died.

While the disease was still raging in Grenada, new cases sprang up in Holly Springs, a small Mississippi community southeast of Memphis, enough so that an epidemic was declared on September 4, sending an already fearful population into a full-scale panic. As in Grenada, the streets were filled with wagons and horses loaded to full capacity as the citizens ran for their lives, many with no idea where they were going.

The citizens who remained took over the Marshall County Courthouse and turned it into a hospital. There were not enough beds available in town to care for the ill, so beds were made of straw and scattered throughout the courthouse. Once they got word of the epidemic, twelve Sisters of Charity from Kentucky traveled to Holly Springs and set up a nursing station in the courthouse.

Clearly frightened by what she saw happening in her town, the wife of the Presbyterian minister wrote: "We seem to dwell in the 'valley of the shadow of death.' . . . I have no one to help me; can get no one. . . . I know you all so feel for us, but you can never know all the painful story, the terrible physical sufferings; those mournful, unattended burials; the sad stillness of death and desolation that prevails. Oh, it is beyond the power of words to describe."[23]

One of Holly Springs's most famous residents, author Katharine Bonner McDowell, who wrote under the pen name of Sherwood Bonner, was in Boston pursuing a writing career to support herself and her young daughter, Lilian, when she received word of the epidemic. Because Lilian had remained in Holly

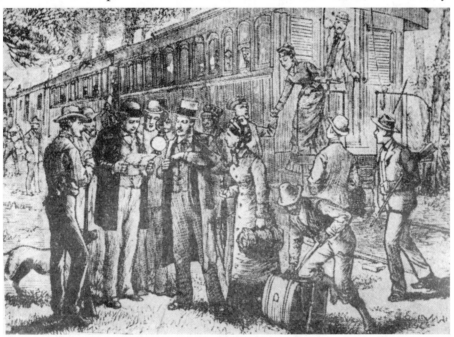

Engraving of men and women boarding a train in Holly Springs, Mississippi, to flee the 1878 yellow fever epidemic.

Springs with Katharine's father and brother (Katharine and her husband were separated), she hurriedly left Boston to go to their aid. Actually, she didn't want to nurse them so much as she wanted to persuade them to join her mother and sisters, who had fled to Kentucky.

What she found when she arrived shocked her to tears. Most of the townspeople had fled, and there was very little activity on the streets. Holly Springs was like a ghost town. On the long train ride south, Katharine corresponded with her good friend, the poet Henry Wadsworth Longfellow, posting letters at stops along the way—and she continued the correspondence after she arrived, expressing her frustration to him. Two days after she reached Holly Springs, both her father and her brother became ill with the fever.

"[Katharine] wired Longfellow about this dire situation on September 4, beseeching, 'Help for God's sake. Send money. Father and brother down [with] yellow fever. [I am] alone to nurse,'" wrote Mississippian historian Deanne Nuwer. "The next day, she again telegraphed Longfellow: 'My heart-breaking. Fear I have the fever.'"[24]

That same day, Katharine's father and brother died of yellow fever, their bodies quickly buried in mass graves with other victims of the plague. Two days later, Katharine broke through the Holly Springs quarantine and returned to Boston, where she completed a novel, *Like unto Like,* which elevated her to the pinnacle of her career. Shortly after that, she divorced her husband on the grounds of abandonment and nonsupport and sent for Lilian, but, within a couple of years, she was diagnosed with breast cancer and returned to Holly Springs, where she compiled, from her deathbed, enough of her already published magazine stories to fill two volumes, *Dialect Tales* and *Suwanee River Tales*, in an effort to provide for Lilian.

Once the epidemic ran its course in Holly Springs, accounts of the town's experiences stayed in the news for many months. One of the lengthier accounts was published in April 1879 by the *Youth's Companion*, a Boston-based weekly magazine that undoubtedly was influenced by Katharine McDowell upon her return to Boston. Calling the town a "pretty, fresh, wholesome place," the magazine told stories of courage and suffering that made "heroes and martyrs" of the people who battled the epidemic.

"A husband lay dying, while at the door, his wife, who had come from a place of safety in the country, begged piteously for admittance," wrote the magazine. "With his dying breath, he said, 'Tell her in all the happy years of our life together, she has never refused to obey a command or request of mine. That is the last I shall make—that she shall not come into my room. Tell her to go home, and live for our children.'"

The greatest admiration expressed by the magazine was directed toward the Sisters of Charity: "Absolutely fearless, cheerful as though walking among flowers in the sunshine, skilled in the arts of nursing, it was a blessed privilege to have them by the sick bed. 'Sister, are you not afraid?' a friend asked one day; 'How can you risk your life for people scarcely known to you by name?' Never shall I forget the look of radiant love that overspread her face, nor the reverent gladness of her tone, as she said: 'It is not the people. I have said 'My God, I offer thee my life. It is Thine to do with as Thou wilt.' This was indeed the spirit that animated all. Out of thirteen [sisters], six laid down their lives, leaving a star-like memory, to brighten always each cherished name."

*   *   *

By 1878 the delta city of Greenville had been to hell and then back again. Burned to the ground by Union troops during the Civil War, it was transformed socially and economically by the Reconstruction years that followed—and then burned to the ground again in 1874 by a fire that began in a downtown warehouse. As the city was rebuilt, African Americans poured into the delta from all over the state to accept sharecropper deals and to work for wages on the sprawling plantations. Even so, there was not enough available labor to all the work that needed to be done. As a result, large numbers of Chinese and Italian immigrants were imported as workers, creating one of the most racially diverse communities in Mississippi.

In 1878 the first yellow fever death in recent memory occurred on August 23, when a four-year-old girl passed away after suffering from a high fever. "While the mother grieved the doctors of the town had met in grave consultation, for near the end there had appeared suspicious symptoms that had caused these wise men much anxiety and fear lest they be dealing for the first time with yellow fever," wrote a young resident of the city, Sue Pelham Trigg. "These physicians . . . had never seen a case of this dread disease, which since June had been raging in New Orleans."[25]

The Greenville death was not announced until August 31, well after panic already had set in a hundred miles away in Grenada. Within one week, there were seventy-five reported cases, with twenty deaths. There had been isolated cases of yellow fever over the years in Greenville, but the city of twenty-five hundred had never experienced an epidemic—and that was one reason the citizens were hit so hard by the one in 1878. For most of its history, the city had existed as an oasis, spared the traumas of many other communities. Now the city knew that it was vulnerable.

Much thought was given to how the little girl could have contracted the disease. Since she had been seen playing on the cotton bales unloaded from New Orleans, some residents thought the disease must reside in cotton. However, discussions about how the little girl had come down with the disease were quickly replaced by fear when it became known that the woman and the nurses who had cared for her also displayed the symptoms of yellow fever. Around that same time, as reported the *Greenville Times*, a group of Chinese immigrants entered the city and had their baggage stored for the night in the railway engine house and then transferred the following day to Stoneville, a small community east of Greenville. Shortly after that, the baggage handler died of yellow fever, along with the brakeman, who had slept in the engine house, and the freight agent.[26]

On September 7, the *Greenville Times* described the progress of the disease: "But eight days have elapsed since yellow fever was declared epidemic in Greenville and during that time 40 deaths have occurred, while 125 cases remain under treatment. No abatement in the disease manifested as yet."[27] A quarantine was quickly instituted, and people were prevented from leaving or entering the city. Ditches were filled with lime, and carbolic acid was scattered on anything that appeared suspicious. Streets were cleaned, and houses were scrubbed and fumigated.

On September 19, the steamer *Ben Allen* pulled into the port at Greenville after being flagged down by frantic residents. After a quick look around the city, the captain sent out a call for help: "Situation is horrible. Four hundred remain and cannot get away; 200 sick; nearly 100 deaths. No boats running; telegraph line down for about ten days; cannot make their wants known; are shut out from the world. For God's sake get nurses, supplies, and money on other boats."[28]

Paranoia was so rampant that armed posses roamed the roads leading into Greenville to bar anyone from entering or leaving the infected city. The telegraph wire was cut, and the posses prevented anyone from repairing it. Finally, in late September, the *Kate Dickson* was filled with provisions in Vicksburg and sent to Greenville, along with a US marshal to oversee repair of the telegraph line.

Trigg, who later published a book about her experiences titled *Recollections of a Little Girl of 1878*, wrote: "There was not a casket left, so they commandeered lumber and men and made plain, unpainted wooden boxes, which served for rich and poor, white and black alike. No longer could the question of family plot in the cemetery be considered. Instead, there was dug grave after grave in long rows, to stand in readiness as the victims fell."

Stevenson Archer, a Greenville minister who contracted yellow fever but recovered, reported that the mayor, the city marshal, and an African American councilman had died of the disease. "Whole families have been swept away, and until the past week we have scarcely well ones enough to hand the sick a drink of water occasionally," he wrote to a fellow minister. "For ten days we were shut up to this horrible sorrow and suffering, but now we have fifty nurses from New Orleans and Vicksburg, and from both points little boats were sent with provisions and medicines, and four physicians. . . . I faced it for twenty days, night and day, from the hut of the pauper to the luxurious apartments of the rich, from the den of the woman of the town to the couch of the holy matron, and I never conceived of such suffering, such ghastly sorrow. I had to succumb then, and for eight days took my turn scorching and tossing, but again am at work."[29]

When the first frost arrived in Greenville in November, there was a celebration. Wrote the *Greenville Times:* "A big white frost last Monday morning was a glorious sight to our people. To those within the affected districts it was a token of rescue and rest; and to those who were shut off from their homes, it was an assurance that their exile would be over, and the sad homecoming at hand."

In December, a memorial service was held in the old opera house on Main Street. Wrote Trigg: "In the center of the building was a massive catafalque, draped heavily in black, symbolic of those graves which lay row on row in the 'God's acre' of the sorrowing little town. . . . All through the service there was a quiet weeping, which broke into heartbroken sobs when 'Paradise, O' Paradise' was sung by Mrs. Walker in her lovely voice so suited to sympathy and comfort."

*   *   *

On January 5, 1879, the Vicksburg *Herald* published a list of the people who had died in Mississippi during the 1878 epidemic, page after page of names—and about a third of them were Vicksburg residents. That month it snowed, allowing people to relax for the first time in more than six months, for they felt that the snow would kill the yellow fever germ, a feeling that was reflected by the newspaper, which wished for snow to also fall in New Orleans. "The yellow fever was no respector of persons," the newspaper observed. "It mowed down the rich and the poor, the good and the bad alike. Whole families were swept away and dear familiar friends were taken in almost countless numbers." That edition of the newspaper also carried a notice from the Howard Association: "Frost having appeared, all persons are requested to thoroughly air all household goods, and ventilate their apartments; and to use disinfect [sic] in cellars and rooms that have been closed during the epidemic."[30]

As the summer of 1879 rolled around, Mississippians took a deep breath. The yellow fever epidemic of 1878 was the worst in American history, and the survivors felt a certain sense of well-being over the fact that they had endured and prevailed. For those inclined to gamble, the odds looked very good, given the sporadic nature of the epidemics that occurred since the Civil War. Most people felt that they would never see another yellow fever epidemic in their lifetime.

That belief was radically altered in September, when a man with yellow fever died near the Illinois central depot in Jackson. Once that news became public, the city panicked. The fever had returned! Businesses closed and people loaded their possessions into wagons and fled. Noted one newspaper, "Everybody was frantically trying to get out, do anything to escape the horrible scourge of yellow fever. Those on the trains were not allowed to stop until they reached Kentucky or Missouri." Edgar Wilson, a correspondent for several out-of-town newspapers, reported: "When yellow fever was announced the people of Jackson arose, like a covey of partridges that was flushed and lit running."

Barely able to contain its own panic, a newspaper calculated from that one known death that one hundred percent of those with the disease had died. Within days of the first death, came news of a second death, prompting a citizen to conclude that "two hundred percent" of the cases had ended in death.

Yellow fever did return to Mississippi and New Orleans in 1879, but it turned out to be a mild visitation, with few deaths. Among those afflicted with the disease was former Confederate general John Bell Hood, a Kentucky-born West Point graduate who saw service at Manassas, Antietam, Gettysburg, Atlanta, and Nashville before surrendering his army to Union forces at Natchez.

After the war, he borrowed $10,000 from friends and took his family to New Orleans, where he founded a business named J. B. Hood and Company, Cotton Factors and Commission Merchants. During his second year in New Orleans, he married Anna Marie Hennen, the daughter of a prominent New Orleans attorney. Hood prospered as a businessman and purchased a large home in the Garden District, which he and his wife proceeded to fill with children, having eleven over a period of ten years—including three sets of twins.

The 1878 epidemic had a devastating effect on Hood, destroying his businesses and forcing him to take his family and flee to Hammond, Louisiana. They weathered the epidemic and returned to New Orleans, where Hood essentially lived off the money he received for mortgaging his house. The following year, when the 1879 epidemic breezed through New Orleans, Mrs. Hood had their eleventh child in July and came down with yellow fever the following month, dying on August 24. Three days later, Hood and his oldest daughter, Lydia, contracted yellow fever. Lydia died on August 29, and Hood died the following day. In 1879 there were only six confirmed deaths resulting from yellow fever in New Orleans, and three of them occurred in the Hood household.

*   *   *

Yellow fever did not appear again in Mississippi until 1897. By late September, there were cases in Vicksburg, Edwards, Biloxi, and Ocean Springs. About the cases in Edwards, the Associated Press reported: "The disease is rapidly spreading and while it is regarded as mild, yet it is feared it will become more malignant, owing to the cool weather now prevailing. We have yet more than a hundred families inside our lines unaffected with a total of about five hundred souls, and indications are that nothing but killing frost will check the disease."[31] The situation became politically inflammatory when the town asked the United States Government to maintain a refugee camp there, only to have authorities, perhaps still fighting imaginary battles left over from the Civil War, denied their request but offered to set up a detention camp. The offer was rejected.

In late September, Jackson mayor Ramsey Wharton boasted that the city had not detected a single case of yellow fever. "Our volunteer policemen are doing the city a fine service, and not a single residence has been broken into or robbed up to this time," he said in a proclamation. "We again urge every citizen to be on the lookout and to report any suspicious person found within our borders. Our police court is now fully installed and anyone found coming into our lines will be punished according to law."

Because there were few cases of yellow fever in Mississippi in October and November, the mood shifted from fear to resentment, as individual towns and cities battled with each other over the quarantine issue. The issued resumed two years later when yellow fever returned for another minor epidemic in September 1899. Jackson mayor Major Porter was one of the first reported cases, and he died shortly after being diagnosed. In all, there were fewer than two dozen cases in Jackson.

In early November, the new mayor, J. W. Todd, issued a proclamation signed by himself and the State Board of Health that was printed in the newspaper under the headline "You Are Invited to Come to Jackson in Safety." The newspaper offered its opinion that the proclamation would "quiet the fears of the outside world": "In view of the lateness of the season the prevailing cold weather and the general conditions now existing, we think it safe for you to return to Jackson. To the traveling public we wish to state that we think there is no danger whatever in you visiting our city, from the fact that there has never been a case of yellow fever in any of the hotels. We respectfully ask all towns in the state to raise their quarantines against us, as we feel absolutely safe in inviting their citizens to come into our community."[32]

CHAPTER FIVE

spanish-american war

finding the real enemy

One year after the devastating yellow fever epidemic of 1878 had run its course in the United States, Dr. Juan Carlos Finlay, then forty-six years of age, was appointed by the Spanish governor of Cuba to work with the United States' National Health Board's Yellow Fever Commission in its efforts to discover how the mysterious disease is transmitted from person to person.

Finlay was no stranger to the island. He was born in Cuba, where he spent his childhood on his father's coffee plantation southwest of Havana. His Scottish-born father was a physician who emigrated as a young man to the West Indies, where he met a woman of French descent living in Trinidad. Once they were married, they moved to Cuba and established the coffee plantation, in addition to starting a family.

When Carlos was eleven, he and his brother Edward were sent to France to be educated. They returned two years later, after Carlos contracted chorea, a disorder that left him with a pronounced stutter. After recovering from chorea, he returned to France to complete his studies, only to come down with a bad case of typhoid. Once again, he went back to Cuba to recover. Instead of returning to France, however, he went to Philadelphia, where he enrolled in Jefferson Medical College. Once he earned his physician's degree in 1855, he considered remaining the United States but found the emotional pull of Cuba too strong to withstand. He set up a practice in Havana in the 1860s and married an Irish woman who, like his mother, was from Trinidad.[1]

At the end of the American Civil War, a handful of Cuban planters freed their slaves, a gesture that led to a ten-year rebellion that saw much fighting between the Spanish overseers and the rebels. In 1878, the final year of the rebellion, yellow fever appeared on the island and was carried north to the United States, possibly instigating the epidemic that devastated the South from New Orleans to Memphis. Intrigued by the mysterious disease, Finlay began studying it in earnest, using the microscope he purchased while in medical school. His appointment to the yellow fever commission the following year opened new doors to him, allowing him to develop a friendship with fellow commission member Dr. George Miller Sternberg.

After a three-month stay in Cuba, the commission concluded that yellow fever was a transmissible disease that was somehow transmitted by airborne agents. Finlay took that conclusion a step further by theorizing that the disease was somehow linked to the blood vessels. In 1881, while attending a conference in Washington, DC, Finlay made a presentation in which he shared his thoughts about how yellow fever was spread. Three ingredients were necessary for the disease to spread, he said—first, there had to be a single case of yellow fever; second, there had to be a susceptible person capable of receiving the disease; and third, there had to be an agent that existed independently of the disease that was capable of transferring the disease from a sick person to a healthy person. He confessed that he didn't know what the transmitting agent was, but he felt certain that if you eliminated that link, you could conquer yellow fever.

Whatever individual members at the conference felt about Finlay's presentation, the report issued after the conference made no mention of his theories. By the time Finlay returned to Cuba, the island had undergone great change. Spain promised to bring about reform in the political and social arenas, prompting celebrations in the streets. Havana was quickly transformed from a staid city, patronized by the planter class, to a wide-open playground controlled by the working class, who preferred exotic Latin rhythms performed by street musicians to opera, brothels to social clubs, and gambling houses to art galleries. It was while those dramatic changes were taking place that the US Yellow Fever Commission issued a report that pointed out the obvious—since 1761, yellow fever had been reported in Havana, not just yearly, but on a monthly basis. From 1856 to 1879, the city had experienced only one month that was, statistically at least, free of the disease.

For the most part, Finlay ignored the social revolution that took place around him, preferring to focus all his efforts on the study of yellow fever. Two years later, in August 1881, Finlay delivered a speech at Havana's Academy of Sciences that set forth his conclusion about the transmission of yellow fever. The culprit, he announced, was the common mosquito. He described the mosquito's anatomy and pointed out how the insect bit humans. Yellow fever, he maintained, was spread when a mosquito bit an infected person and then carried it to the next human it bit. He admitted that he had no scientific proof.

Finlay was never able to adequately explain how he arrived at his mosquito theory, but his work may have been influenced by the earlier research of Patrick Manson, who discovered that filariasis, a disfiguring disease sometimes called elephantiasis, was transmitted by mosquitoes. Manson arrived at that decision after conducting experiments with mosquitoes, using individuals with contaminated blood.[2]

When Finlay finished his speech, the audience looked at him in stunned silence. It was the craziest thing they had ever heard. They didn't even bother to applaud when he turned to sit down. Behind his back, they called him a crazy old man. Finlay was hurt by the rejection of his ideas, but he did not curtail his research. He moved his office to a remote part of the island that had reported no yellow fever cases in more than a decade. There he set out to prove a connection between the mosquito and the disease. Over the next thirteen years, he inoculated almost one hundred human subjects, producing twelve cases that he diagnosed as yellow fever. Only one of those cases stood up to scrutiny, however—the other subjects showed symptoms too mild to be definitive. Undeterred, Finlay attended a medical conference in Budapest in 1894, at which he called for the eradication of the mosquito. Again, his suggestions were ignored.

Paralleling the work done by Carlos Finlay in the late 1880s was that done by Finlay's friend, Dr. George Sternberg. Sternberg was born and educated in New York, where his father was on the faculty at Harwick Seminary. Shortly after George Sternberg received his medical degree from the College of Physicians and Surgeons in New York City, the Civil War began, inspiring him to join the Union Army. He was captured at the battle of Bull Run, but he escaped after a brief detention and made his way back to Washington, DC, where he remained. After the war, he stayed in the army and treated soldiers wounded in the Indian wars. It was while serving as a US Army physician that Sternberg began his self-taught research in bacteriology, becoming the first researcher to identify a bacterium as a cause of pneumonia and the first to discover parasites in the blood of malaria patients.

Yellow fever was high on his list of mysteries to solve. His first medical paper, "An Inquiry into the Modus Operandi of the Yellow Fever Poison," was published in 1875 in the *New Orleans Medical and Surgical Journal*. By the time he went to Cuba to serve on the commission with Carlos Finlay, he had gained a reputation as the leading authority on yellow fever in the US Army. Although the commission failed in its efforts to find a cause of yellow fever, the experience did encourage Sternberg to continue his own private research.

In late 1877 and early 1888, Finlay sent Sternberg mosquito cultures that contained clusters of bacteria that Finlay thought could be the yellow fever germ. Sternberg studied the cultures but reported that, while the bacteria were often found in association with yellow fever, they were not the cause of the disease. In 1888 Sternberg heard from a French physician in Havana who claimed to have isolated the yellow fever germ. He went to Havana to investigate but decided it was a false alarm. The following year, he returned to Cuba to observe an epidemic.

In 1890 Sternberg published a book about yellow fever in which he concluded that the disease was the result of a micro-organism. He linked it to typhoid and cholera, though he admitted that it did not follow the transmission patterns associated with those diseases. His only major recommendation was that the bodily fluids associated with yellow fever—black vomit, feces, urine, and blood—should be viewed as infectious material that requires disinfecting before it is disposed of. Two years later, he published a textbook on bacteriology that established him as the leading expert on the subject.

Primarily because of his celebrity, Sternberg was named surgeon general of the US Army in 1893. One of his first major accomplishments was the creation of the Army Medical School in Washington, DC. It was not a medical school in the strict sense—that is, it did not teach primary medicine to inexperienced students—but rather it taught graduates of civilian medical schools how to practice army medicine.

One of the first officers to report to duty at the school was Captain Walter Reed, who was asked to be the curator of the Army Medical Museum in addition to his duties at the new medical school. Born in Virginia ten years before the start of the Civil War, Reed saw two of his brothers serve with the Confederacy. Both brothers survived, but one returned with an amputated hand, having reportedly told the surgeon after the surgery, "Thank you, doctor, you have left me enough to hang the girls on." During the war, Walter Reed and another brother hid the family's horses when they heard that General Philip Sheridan's men were in the area looking for horses to steal. The boys were picked up by the soldiers and briefly held—and the horses were taken from them anyway.[3]

After the war, Reed enrolled at the University of Virginia at the age of fifteen in the hope of obtaining a master's degree. However, since the degree requirements were more time-consuming and costly than he anticipated, he transferred to the medical school at the age of seventeen. At that time, it was much easier to get a medical degree than it was to get a master's degree primarily because being a physician was not considered a real profession by many people. After spending nine months studying to become a physician, he was graduated third in his class, the youngest student at the university ever to graduate in medicine.

With his degree in hand, Reed went to New York's Bellevue Hospital to gain clinical experience. While at the hospital to earn an MD degree, he applied for the position of assistant physician at the Infants' Hospital at Randall's Island. He ranked first on the exam and was given the position. Although he had finished his work at Bellevue, the hospital withheld his degree until he turned twenty-one.

For the next five years, Reed went through a series of positions—first, at Kings County Hospital in Brooklyn and then as assistant sanitary officer at the Brooklyn Board of Health. It was during that time that he became disillusioned with medicine. All around him, physicians without diagnostic skills used crude treatments such as bleeding to treat patients who obviously needed alternative medical care. One day, a wealthy physician who was dressed in the latest fashion filed a report with Reed regarding the death of an infant. The report was so ignorant, complete with misspellings, that Reed angrily informed his family that he was ready to leave medicine and pursue another career.

In despair of his chosen profession—and with his nerves on

edge—Reed got into a fight with a German boarder in his rooming house over a perceived insult, one that Reed argued would justify a duel in his home state of Virginia. To his disappointment, both his landlady and his boss sided with the German. A year later, he went to visit his family and met a young girl named Emilee Lawrence in church. During their courtship, the twenty-four-year-old decided to apply for a position in the US Army, a decision that quickly saw his appointment as an assistant surgeon and first lieutenant.

Reed pursued Emilee with the same zeal he applied to his career, but he found her to be in no hurry to commit her heart. Unable to persuade her in person, he sent her letters that expressed his feelings. In one letter, he wrote: "During the past 6 years I have seen something of the affection which men and women bear toward one another; (God knows, I must confess that I have witnessed its absence more than its presence;) . . . during these years I have given much thought to this subject . . . living in the largest city in America, I have seen & met the most fascinating women; and yet need I tell you & *you alone* are the only woman whom I have admired."[4] Reed entered the army without winning Emilee's hand, but, after a series of frustrating military assignments, he finally succeeded in winning her heart, and they were married on April 26, 1876.

For nearly two decades, Reed worked at building both a family and an army career. He was transferred many times, from Nebraska to Maryland to New York to Alabama, assignments that allowed him to rise to the rank of captain but did little to further his studies as a physician. It was not until October 1890 that he got the break he had hoped for and was allowed to take postgraduate courses in pathology and bacteriology at Johns Hopkins Hospital. When he heard of George Sternberg's appointment as surgeon general, he wrote a congratulatory note: "It places at the head of the Corps the one man who preeminently stands forth as the representative of progressive scientific medicine. . . . The fossil age has passed."[5] Sternberg was impressed enough with Reed to take him under his wing at his new school and to actively promote his career as a physician.

By that point, all the players but one were in place for the medical profession's showdown with yellow fever in Cuba. The fourth player was William Gorgas, an Alabama-born "army brat" who grew up moving from place to place as his father pursued a career in the US Army. When he was seven, his father was put in charge of the armory at Charleston, South Carolina—a fortuitous event that allowed him and his sister to sit on the porch of their home and hear the guns at Fort Sumter as the opening shots in the Civil War were fired. His father resigned his commission with the army and joined the Confederacy, after which he was commissioned a brigadier general and put in charge of the ordnance for the Confederacy.

Gorgas grew into adulthood with memories of the war and of the poverty that his parents faced after the war. When he was of age, he applied for admission to the United States Military Academy so that he could follow in his father's footsteps, but his applications—and there were several—were always rejected for a variety of reasons. Finally, he figured out that if he went to medical school and got a degree, the army would give him a commission. In 1876, at the age of twenty-two, Gorgas entered Bellevue Medical College in New York, finally earning his degree as a doctor of medicine in 1879. Then, as planned, he entered the medical corps of the US Army a few months later. He was assigned to an infantry company and ordered to avoid any contact with yellow fever patients. When he disobeyed the order and entered the yellow fever ward of the post hospital, he was promptly arrested and confined to quarters. However, when the division commander was advised of his arrest, he quickly ordered Gorgas released.

As the years went by, Gorgas was recognized as an expert on yellow fever. Typically, he was summoned each time an outbreak was identified. When the disease appeared at Fort Barrancas, Florida, he was sent there to do what he could to treat the sick. In addition to providing medical treatment, he was asked to dig graves, wrap the dead in shrouds, and conduct the religious service once the grave was filled in.

So there you have it—Finlay, Sternberg, Reed, and Gorgas were poised on the brink of greatness when the Spanish-American War exploded in their faces and threw everything up into the air.

*   *   *

By 1895 it was obvious to Cuban workers that the reforms promised by Spain would never take place. Slavery was abolished in 1886, as promised, but working conditions on the island were not significantly improved. As a result, two Cuban generals, Bartolome Maso and Maximo Gomez, initiated a insurrection against Spain that brought about a strong response. Spanish authorities established interrogation camps, similar to the one the United States would build more than one hundred years later to house prisoners from the Iraq and Afghanistan wars, and herded women and children into them, where many died of starvation. The rebels responded by destroying the cane fields and sugar mills owned by Spanish investors.

American businessmen, eager to acquire interests in the sugar plantations, urged US President William McKinley to join the war on the side of the rebels, but he was reluctant to do so. Instead, he offered to mediate a peaceful solution between Spain and the rebels. It was a slow process, but it seemed to bear fruit two years later when Spain removed its most hated general and promised to give its colony some form of self-rule. Throughout the mediation process, American military ships docked in Cuban harbors without incident to take on supplies.

Opposed to McKinley's approach were Cuban refugees in Florida and the businessmen who supported an extension of the government's "manifest destiny" doctrine, which, simply put, declared that the United States had a claim to all the land on the continent between Canada and Mexico. Not satisfied with "manifest destiny" being applied solely to the continental land area, American corporations wanted to see the United States become an imperial power along the lines of Great Britain. They argued that the United States should expand into the seas and beyond. Basically, the proponents of expansion were descendants of the same wealthy families that were against the Revolutionary War. All those years later, they wanted to remake America in the image of England—and Cuba seemed like an excellent first step.

Waging an intense propaganda war against Spain during that time was newspaper publisher William Randolph Hearst, whose chain of newspapers reached into almost every city in the United States. Hearst was the son of a wealthy mine owner and former US senator from California who dabbled in politics. The young Hearst was sent to Harvard University, where he edited the *Harvard Lampoon*. Upon graduation he was given his first newspaper, the *San Francisco Examiner*, which he used as a platform to build his newspaper empire and to express his peculiar vision of journalism, later dubbed "yellow journalism." To Hearst, a newspaper was an extension of the political process. He used news stories, which were often exaggerated to the point of becoming outright fiction, to shape public opinion on issues he felt were important.

In January 1897, while President McKinley was pursuing a diplomatic strategy, Hearst sent an illustrator/correspondent named Frederick Remington to Cuba to report on the great battles reportedly taking place between the Spanish and the Cubans. When Remington learned that none of the battles that Hearst newspapers had been reporting were actually taking place, he cabled his employer: "Everything is quiet. There is no trouble. There will be no war. I wish to return." Although Hearst later denied it, Remington said that his boss quickly wired back: "Please remain. You furnish the pictures and I'll furnish the war."

One year later, on January 25, 1898, the *USS Maine*, a second-class battleship that was as long as a football field, entered Havana harbor at the request of the American consul who sought its presence to protect American interests. Its captain, Charles Sigsbee, entertained Spanish officers aboard the ship and allowed his crewmen to be entertained by local officials. After a three-week stay, Sigsbee was optimistic about the situation in Cuba. The city was peaceful, and he saw no sign of rebel activity.

That sense of well-being quickly changed on the evening of February 15 with a tremendous explosion. Sigsbee had just finished writing a letter when it happened. "It was a bursting, rending, and crashing roar of immense volume, largely metallic in character," he wrote. "There was a trembling and lurching motion of the vessel, a list to port. The lights went out. Then there was intense blackness and smoke."

The forward portion of the ship sank quickly, killing 254 seamen and wounding fifty-nine others. Under the headline "The Maine Blown Up," the *New York Times* reported:

> As yet the cause of the explosion is not apparent. The wounded sailors of the Maine are unable to explain it. It is believed that the battleship is totally destroyed. The explosion shook the whole city. The windows were broken in nearly all the houses. . . . Senor de Lome, the departing ex-Minister of Spain to this country, who arrived in this city last night, and went to the Hotel St. Marc, at Fifth Avenue and Thirty-ninth Street, was awakened on the receipt of the news from Havana. He refused to believe the report at first. When he had been assured of the truth of the story he said that there was no possibility that the Spaniards had anything to do with the destruction of the Maine. No Spaniard, he said would be guilty of such an act. If the report was true, he said, the explosion must have been caused by some accident on board the warship.[6]

The ship's sinking was reported differently by Hearst's *New York Journal,* which published illustrations of how Spanish terror-

ists fastened an underwater mine to the *Maine* and then deto-
nated it from shore. Day after day, week after week, Hearst's newspapers, using headlines such as "Remember the Maine," beat the
drums for war with Spain. Soon the newspapers were joined by
businesses that envisioned huge economic gains in Cuba, and
together they demanded that America's honor be avenged.

Several years later, Hearst correspondent James Creelman
wrote in his memoirs that he was proud of his boss for the way he
promoted the war. In defense of Hearst's so-called yellow journalism, Creelman wrote: "[It] deserves its place among the most
useful instrumentalities of civilization. It may be guilty of giving
the world a lop-sided view of events by exaggerating the importance of a few things and ignoring others, it may offend the eye
by typographical violence, it may sometimes proclaim its own
deeds too loudly; but it never deserted the cause of the poor and
downtrodden."

The effect of that type of journalism—or antijournalism, as
most journalists would call it today—was felt for decades to come.
An American history book, published in 1917 for student use,
used similar language, emotional to the ear and void of facts, in
its chapter on the Spanish-American War. About the *USS Maine,* it
wrote: "Instantly the people were aroused. They demanded war."

Spain offered to submit the *Maine* incident to international
arbitration, and the Spanish government demanded an end to
fighting in Cuba, but that was not enough for the US government, which was beginning to feel pressure to take action. The
president ordered a naval blockade of Havana and the northern
coast of the island, and Commodore George Dewey was ordered
to take his fleet to the Philippines, which also was owned by
Spain. Meanwhile, Congress gave the president the authority to
use the army and navy to force the Spanish off the island—and
finally declared war on Spain on April 21, 1898.

American expansionists like Hearst were delighted. The *Maine*
not only provided the United States with an excuse to seize Cuba

but also made it possible for an American takeover of the Philippines, Guam, and Puerto Rico, an obvious financial bonanza to American businesses interested in exploiting the islands' natural resources.

America's battle plan was twofold—Commodore Dewey was ordered to defeat the Spanish fleet at Manila, and naval and ground forces were ordered to defeat the Spanish fleet at Santiago by mounting a pincher attack. Among those charged with winning ground victories was Lieutenant Colonel Theodore Roosevelt, commander of the famous Roughriders regiment.

Amazingly, American military planners scheduled their heaviest activities for July and August, when yellow fever on the island was at its peak. No one knows what they were thinking, for it was well known that Cuba experienced epidemics every summer. With the outbreak of the war, Dr. William Gorgas was sent to Cuba, where he quickly befriended Dr. Carlos Finlay.

Gorgas did not believe Finlay's theory about mosquitoes being an agent for the transmission of yellow fever, but he had great respect for the old doctor and valued his friendship. Nothing should be read into Gorgas's transfer to the island, insofar as his expertise about yellow fever was concerned, because all available medical personnel were sent. At that time, the Army Medical Corps had only 177 commissioned officers and 750 enlisted men to care for the entire army. Additional physicians were hastily recruited from the private sector, many of them incompetent, a decision that was not greeted with enthusiasm among rank-and-file army physicians.

Apparently, the only consideration military planners gave to yellow fever was the decision to send the Twenty-fourth and Twenty-fifth Infantries to Cuba. Since they were all-black regiments, it was felt that they possessed a special immunity to the disease. We have a record of their service in Cuba because the African American chaplain of the Twenty-fifth Infantry, Theophilus G. Steward, wrote about their experiences in a book titled *The Colored*

Regulars in the United States Army.[7] The Twenty-fifth Infantry's first combat service occurred at the battle of El Caney, which saw them charge up the hill with great gallantry, so much so that, as the regiment came back down the hill after the battle, the soldiers were applauded and cheered by the Second Massachusetts Volunteers. Later, the Twenty-fifth Infantry linked with the Twenty-fourth Infantry on the outskirts Santiago, where they dug in and held a trench line until the end of the war.

The deaths of so many officers from the Twenty-fourth and Twenty-fifth Infantries promoted the racist theory that the officers of black troops were required to expose themselves to a greater degree of fighting than their white counterparts in order to lead their hesitant men. Not so, wrote Steward, who quoted a captain: "The gallantry and bearing shown by the officers and soldiers of the regiment under this trying ordeal was such that it has every reason to be proud of its record. The losses of the regiment, which are shown by the official records, show the fire they were subjected to. The casualties were greater among the officers than the men, which is accounted for by the fact that the enemy had posted in the trees sharpshooters, whose principal business was to pick them off."

As it turned out, Spanish sharpshooters were not the real enemy. In skirmish after skirmish, the Spanish were defeated in quick order, with American forces sustaining relatively light casualties. The enemy that took down the most American soldiers was yellow fever. Immediately after the victory at Santiago on July 3, army leaders asked Secretary of War Russell Alger to allow the army to move to higher ground, away from the city. In a letter to Alger, Lieutenant Colonel Theodore Roosevelt encouraged Alger to take action: "If we are kept here it will in all human possibility mean an appalling disaster, for the surgeons here estimate that over half the army, if kept here during the sickly season, will die." By the time Roosevelt wrote the letter, two thousand soldiers already were infected with yellow fever.

Alger held his ground, or rather ordered the soldiers to hold their ground, until the Spanish forces in Santiago surrendered. On July 15, two days before the city's surrender, word arrived at the Twenty-fourth that a large hospital had been set up at Siboney. Later that day, the regiment was ordered to proceed to Siboney and report to its medical officer. By the end of the day, the regiment, consisting of eight companies containing fifteen officers and 456 men, had marched through the night, arriving at Siboney at 3:30 in the morning. Not until they arrived did the men learn that their assignment was to care for the growing number of yellow fever patients.

"On the day of arrival seventy men were called for to nurse yellow fever patients and do other work about the hospital," wrote Steward. "More than this number immediately volunteered to enter upon a service which they could well believe meant death to some of them. The camp was so crowded and filthy that the work of cleaning it was begun at once by the men of the Twenty-fourth, and day by day they labored as their strength would permit, in policing the camp, cooking the food for themselves and for the hospital, unloading supplies, taking down and removing tents, and numberless other details of necessary labor."

Out of the 456 men who went to Siboney, reported Steward, only twenty-four failed to come down with the disease—and, at one point, 241 men in the Twenty-fourth were ill on a single day. "Those who would recover remained weak and unfit for labor," Steward wrote. "Silently, without murmuring, did these noble heroes, officers and men, stand at their post ministering to the necessities of their fellowmen until the welcome news came that the regiment would be sent north and the hospital closed as soon as possible." When the Twenty-fourth was allowed to leave Siboney on August 26, it marched out of the camp with it colors flying and its band playing, despite the fact that it left 198 men behind, casualties of yellow fever.

In the interim, between the surrender of Santiago in July and the signing of the Treaty of Paris on December 10, 1898, the American fleet occupied the Spanish island of Puerto Rico so that, when the time came to work out the details of the treaty, America was in position to ask for Cuba's independence and to take control of the colonies of Puerto Rico, the Philippines, and Guam. The treaty, which gave the United States complete control of the Caribbean Sea and provided it with a stepping stone to Asian markets, made America a colonial power, thus realizing some Americans' long-held dreams of becoming closet monarchists. It was the first war fought for the benefit of American corporations, but not the last, as experiences in Vietnam and Iraq would later demonstrate.

Although American leaders later denied that corporations influenced their decision to go to war—and everyone from the president down voiced a desire to remove American influence from the island as soon as possible so that Cubans could determine their own future—it quickly became evident that would not be the case. Soon, half of Cuba's farmland was taken over by American corporations in an effort to take control of the entire sugar industry. Americans were appointed to govern the island, and they were backed by an occupation force whose main assignment was to protect American corporate interests. American military forces finally left in 1909, but not before forcing Cuba to lease its land for a naval base at Guantanamo Bay.

The Spanish-American War was costly for many reasons. Only 968 American soldiers were lost to hostile fire, but more than five thousand died of yellow fever, a devastating loss to America's relatively small army. America's position in the international community was lowered a notch by the war because other nations became suspicious of America's long-range intentions. And, finally, the war created fears among American citizens that government leaders had a secret agenda to expand American influence all over the globe—and that was not a position supported by most Americans.

Perhaps for that reason, the Spanish-American War remained

a nagging thorn in American foreign policy for many years, with questions repeatedly asked about the country's justification for going to war. Many years later, Admiral Hyman G. Rickover continued the debate with a book published in 1979 titled *How the Battleship Maine Was Destroyed*. Before writing the book, Rickover assembled a team of experts to see whether they could determine the origins of the explosion that sank the *USS Maine*. They concluded that the most likely cause for the explosion was spontaneous combustion associated with coal in the bunker next to the ammunition magazine. Rickover's report was greeted with varying degrees of enthusiasm by those opposed to the war, ridicule from those who supported the war, and hostility from those who felt that the admiral's "solution" was a cover-up to protect American businessmen thought to be responsible for the blast—and, after a century of scrutiny, the mystery remains unresolved.

*   *   *

In the wake of the Spanish-American War, while American troops were still stationed in Cuba as occupation forces and being subjected to relentless attacks of both typhoid and yellow fever, Surgeon General Sternberg became concerned about the possible transfer of typhoid to the mainland by returning troops. He called on Walter Reed, along with E. O. Shakespeare and Victor Vaughan—all three of whom served on the typhoid board—to find out what was happening in the camps.

The board traveled from camp to camp, where they examined patients and inspected wells—and pored over travel records so that they could account for the whereabouts of each soldier and the routes each man took to get to the camps. They were discouraged by what they found: The medical corps was in shambles, led by physicians who had little understanding of infectious diseases and even less understanding of the importance of keeping detailed and accurate records on each patient in their care.

Before the board could issue a report of its findings, Reed was ordered to take on a new project—determining whether a big resort hotel at Natural Bridge, Virginia, could be converted into a military hospital. In Reed's absence, Shakespeare and Vaughan continued but were discharged from the army in June 1899 as part of an economic cutback. Unfortunately, Shakespeare died before the report could be written. Luckily, Reed had written an abstract of their proposed report, leaving Vaughan to put together a more extensive analysis of their findings. When Vaughan's paper was published, there was no mention of the contributions made by Reed and Shakespeare.

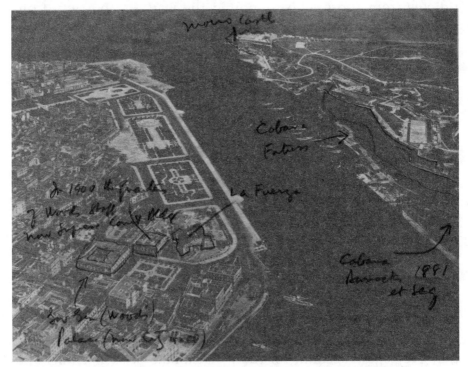

Aerial view of Havana with sites marked by Philip Hench.

By that time, Sternberg had already put together a commission to investigate the disturbing situation in Cuba. Reed was appointed its presiding officer. Also on the yellow fever board were Reed's assistant, Canadian bacteriologist James Carroll, and two men already in Cuba, Jesse Lazear, a bacteriologist from Johns Hopkins Hospital, and Cuban-born Aristides Agramonte, a member of the Army Medical Corps. Of the four men, only Agramonte had survived yellow fever as a child and therefore acquired immunity to the disease. Since none of the other three men had immunity, they knew they risked their lives by working with yellow fever patients.[8]

Reed and Carroll sailed from New York to Havana on the first day of summer, and by early July they had the yellow fever board in operation. One of their nurses was Lena Warner, the daughter of a prominent Mississippi family. She had firsthand knowledge of yellow fever. Not only did the 1878 epidemic kill her father and several other family members in Grenada, but also it left her ill with the disease. She survived and spent the remainder of her childhood with her grandmother, but she never forgot the terror she experienced living through a yellow fever epidemic. It was probably the reason she decided to become a nurse. Immediately after she was graduated from Tennessee's first nursing program (she was the program's first student), she enrolled in the teaching program at Cook County Hospital in Chicago for postgraduate study in surgery. Not long after she returned to Memphis to be hired as an assistant at the School of Nursing, she saw a newspaper advertisement soliciting immune nurses to serve in Cuba.[9]

Warner arrived in Cuba three months before the yellow fever board went into operation. She was appointed chief nurse at the hospital at Matanzas and put in charge of the fever tents, where she worked until Reed and his board members arrived, at which time she was ordered to Columbia Barracks, six miles outside Havana.

One of the first things that Reed did upon arriving in Cuba was to visit his old friend Jefferson Randolph Kean, a career medical officer who had come down with yellow fever. Reed was eager to see his friend, not just because of their past associations, but because Kean was in the early stages of the disease—and Reed had never seen an actual case of yellow fever. Kean offered his opinion

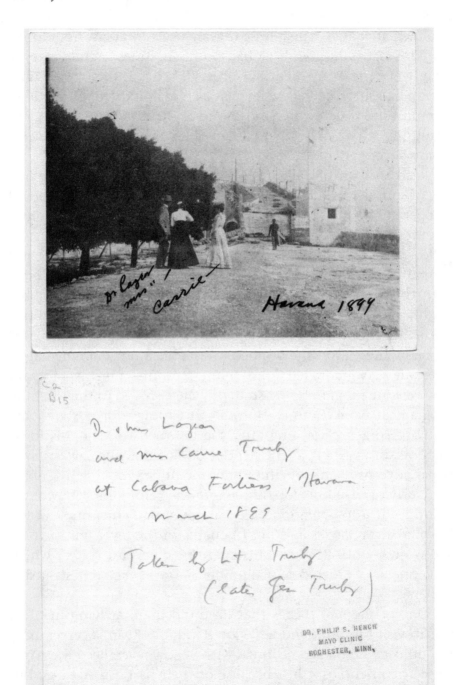

Jesse W. Lazear, Mabel Lazear, and Carrie Truby in Havana.

that the Cuban habit of doing laundry in previously used water might contribute to the spread of the disease. He also suggested that Cuban whorehouses could also play a role.

As it turned out, Kean's infection was because of neither dirty laundry nor to a visit to a whorehouse, but rather to compassion for his fellow officers infected with the disease. He was a frequent visitor to Columbia Barracks, where yellow fever cases were isolated from the general population. When his superiors learned of this, they ordered him to terminate his visits as long as he was working in headquarters. He obeyed the order, but, when a close friend came down with the disease and was moved to Columbia Barracks, Kean decided to pay him a visit. "I was too much worried about him to sleep," Kean later wrote, "and so arose at daybreak on the sixteenth of June and went over to his house. There I complied with . . . [the] order by sitting on the porch and talking through the window, which was closed only with an iron grill."[10] Five days later, Kean came down with yellow fever.

Reed left his friend's bedside feeling that Kean's attack was a mild one and that he had a good chance for recovery. Later, Reed and the other board members called on Carlos Finlay. No one in their group was convinced that Finlay's mosquito theory was the answer, but they wanted to consider every possibility. Finlay was delighted to see them and presented them with a gift of eggs from a mosquito that he was certain had transmitted yellow fever. He told them that if they placed the eggs in water, a larva would appear in three days, and an adult mosquito would hatch in about a week and a half. Finlay had no explanation for how the disease could be passed from mosquito to egg to larvae to human, just a hunch that something important took place during that process.

Back at their testing facility, Lazear took charge of the mosquito eggs and, following Finlay's instructions, carefully hatched them and put each mosquito in a separate test tube. Meanwhile, Reed and the other board members devised a plan to test Finlay's theory on human subjects. They all agreed that, in the best interests of science, at least from an ethical standpoint, they should expose themselves to whatever tests they used on human subjects. In addition to themselves, they sought volunteers from American soldiers and Spanish immigrants, two groups they felt would not have acquired immunity to the disease. The consent form was brief and to the point: "The undersigned understands perfectly well that in the case of the development of yellow fever in him, that he endangers his life to a certain extent but it being entirely impossible for him to avoid the infection during his stay on this island he prefers to take the chance of contracting it intentionally in the belief that he will receive from the said Commission the greatest care and the most skillful medical service."[11]

Volunteers were offered one hundred dollars in gold for their services, payable at the conclusion of the experiment. In the event they contracted yellow fever as a result of the experiment, they would be paid an additional one hundred dollars, a payment that was guaranteed to be passed on to their beneficiary in the event of their death.

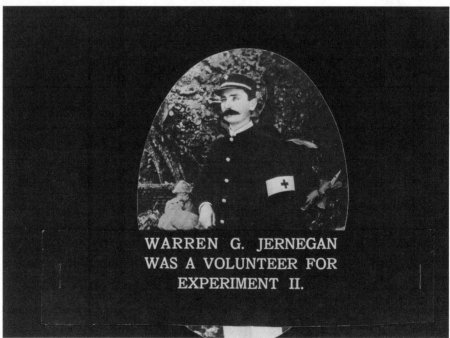

WARREN G. JERNEGAN
WAS A VOLUNTEER FOR
EXPERIMENT II.

Warren Jernegan, yellow fever volunteer.

Lazear's method of using the volunteers was relatively simple, dependent only on his ability to keep the insects alive long enough to be used in the experiments: Individual tubes of mosquitoes were taken to a hospital where yellow fever patients were being cared for, and they were exposed to the mosquitoes by uncorking the test tubes and pressing the open end on the flesh of the patient, allowing the mosquito unfettered access to the patients' blood supply. The infected mosquitoes were then taken to their laboratory, where they were allowed, using the same procedure, to feed on the volunteers.

Lazear allowed himself to be bitten on August 16, 1900, by one of the infected insects. When he did not develop the disease within a reasonable time, he placed an infected insect on Dr. James Carroll's arm. This time the experiment was successful. Within four days, Carroll, who never believed that mosquitoes carried the disease, showed all the symptoms of yellow fever. Once he realized he was ill, he sent for his friend, Dr. William Gorgas, who promptly diagnosed him as having yellow fever. Gorgas asked nurse Lena Warner, who worked under Gorgas's supervision, to take care of his friend Carroll. "Major Gorgas was very successful in the treatment of the fever," she later wrote, "I determined to imitate his directions."[12]

By September 13, Carroll's recovery seemed certain. On that day, Lazear was collecting blood samples from yellow fever patients at the hospital when he noticed a mosquito land on the back of his hand. Not wishing to abort the medical procedure in order to kill the mosquito, he allowed the insect to feed on his blood until it was satiated and flew away. Five days later, while Carroll was leaving the hospital, Lazear complained of a chill, and, the following day, he had a temperature of 102.4 degrees and a pulse rate of 112. Jaundice appeared on the third day, and his temperature went over 103 degrees. He died on the sixth day. The *Chicago Record* reported his passing with a story that ran under the headline "Dr. Lazear Really Sacrificed His Life to Science": "The recent death in Cuba of Dr. Jesse Lazear, caused by an attack of yellow fever, furnishes a pathetic and interesting example of one among a limited few who have really sacrificed themselves to science. . . . Working early and late in a climate to which he was unused and which was swarming with the germs he was studying, it is not strange that he himself fell an easy prey to the ravages of the dreaded bacillus."[13]

The newspaper's use of the phrase "dreaded bacillus" was indicative of the scientific community's view of the disease. Surgeon General Sternberg had always felt that the disease was caused by bacteria, his approval of the mosquito experiments notwithstanding. Even Walter Reed seemed to lean in that direction, though he felt that the mosquito was the vehicle through which the bacillus was transmitted. Ironically, it was Lazear who had no faith in the bacillus theory and a great deal of faith in the mosquito.

Reed, who was in the States at the time of Lazear's death, presented a paper, "Some Observations on the Yellow Fever in Cuba," at a meeting of the American Public Health Association. The paper, which identified the mosquito as the host for a "parasite" that caused yellow fever, was received with indifference by the group. Reed left a copy of the paper with his boss, Surgeon General Sternberg, and did not think much about it until later, when he learned that Sternberg had arranged for its publication in the *Philadelphia Medical Journal*. Retitled "The Etiology of Yellow Fever: A Preliminary Note," it cited Reed as author, with Carroll, Agramonte, and Lazear as contributing editors. Reed wrote: "Since we have here, for the first time, record of a case in which a typical attack of yellow fever has followed the bite of an infected mosquito, within the usual period of incubation of the disease, and in which other sources of infection can be excluded, we feel confident that the publication of those observations must excite renewed interest in the mosquito theory of the propagation of yellow fever, as first proposed by Finlay."

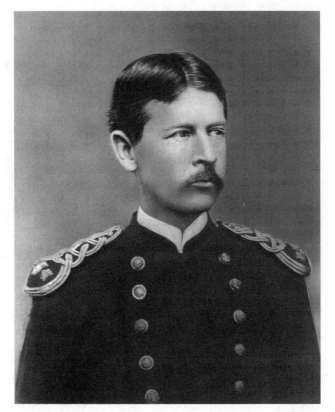

Major Walter Reed.

To Reed's dismay, reaction to the article was mixed. The *Washington Post* described his theory as silly. However, the *New York Times* took Reed's theory more seriously: "As Dr. Lazear was bitten by a mosquito while present in the wards of a yellow fever hospital, one must, at least, admit the possibility of this insect's contamination by a previous bite of a yellow fever patient. This case of accidental infection therefore cannot fail to be of interest."[14]

Because of the criticism he received for his research, Reed made plans to return to Cuba, determined to repeat the experiments in a more controlled setting calculated to silence his critics. Lazear's death had been the result of a random encounter with a mosquito and proved nothing, at least from a scientific perspective. Carroll's death was in much the same category. Yes, Lazear had placed a mosquito on his arm, but Reed did not feel that it

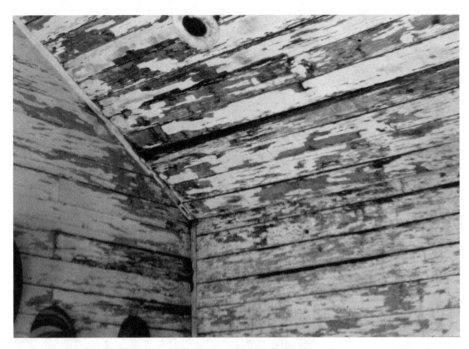

Interior of Building No. 1, Camp Lazear.

was not done under the sort of controlled situation that would withstand scientific scrutiny.

Before leaving the States, Reed wrote Carroll a letter congratulating him on his speedy recovery, adding, "I shall simply go out and get boiling drunk! Really I can never recall such a sense of relief in all my life, as the news of your recovery gives me!" On the back of the envelope, he wrote, "Did the mosquito do it?"

Reed arrived in Cuba on October 4 and quickly reorganized his project, moving the experimental camp one mile away from Columbia Barracks to a new location he named Camp Lazear. Of the original four members of the yellow fever board, only Reed and Carroll remained. Lazear had died, and Agramonte was in the States on leave. Not long after Reed arrived, Carroll went home on sick leave.

Certainly, Carroll was justified in taking leave, but comments he wrote in letters shortly after Reed's arrival suggest he may have had other reasons. Carroll stated that a military officer had commented on Reed's absence by saying, "I think I shall have to accuse him of running away." In a letter to his wife, Carroll wrote: "My friend [Reed] will be as brave as a lion now that the yellow fever season is about over and he will take particular care not to take the same chances I did. . . . I will never get [recognition] as long as it is in my friends' [sic] power to prevent it."[15]

Working alone, Reed gathered up Lazear's notebooks and proceeded at a frenetic pace that no one who knew him had ever seen. Usually, he was slow and studied, deliberate in his actions and thought process, always willing to discuss his work. The new Walter Reed was hyperactive and prone to secrecy—and just a bit paranoid. It surprised no one when he placed an armed guard around Camp Lazear. A hospital steward who had acquired immunity to the disease was asked to bring supplies from Camp Columbia, but no other contact with the outside world was permitted to those who worked in the camp as medical personnel or volunteers.

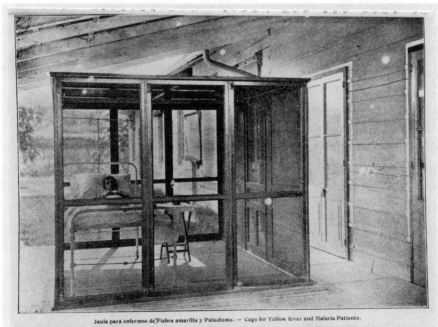

Jaula para enfermos de Fiebre amarilla y Paludismo. — Cage for Yellow fever and Malaria Patients.

Cage for yellow fever patients, Havana.

In one experiment, Reed exposed volunteers to the soiled clothing and bedding of patients who had died of yellow fever. Reed described the experiment in his paper, "The Etiology of Yellow Fever": "The majority of the articles had been taken from the beds of patients sick with yellow fever at Las Animas Hospital, Havana, or at Columbia Barracks. Many of them had been purposely soiled with a liberal quantity of black vomit, urine and fecal matter. A dirty 'comfortable' [sic] and much soiled pair of blankets, removed from a bed of a patient sick with yellow fever in the town of Quemados, were contained in these boxes."

Since no cases of yellow fever were reported as a result of that exposure, Reed concluded that contaminated clothing could not transmit the disease. That experiment seemed to be done for the benefit of Surgeon General Sternberg and others who thought that bacteria were involved in the transmission of the disease. In another experiment, a frame building was constructed and screened to prevent mosquitoes from entering or leaving. The interior was divided into two compartments, separated by wire netting. Two men without immunity were placed into one side, and one man without immunity was placed into the other side.

After the men remained there for several days, Reed placed fifteen yellow fever–bearing mosquitoes into the compartment occupied by one man, and he was allowed to be bitten several times by the mosquitoes. Four days later, he came down with yellow fever. The two men who lived in the other compartment remained healthy, despite breathing the same air. Reed then removed the infected mosquitoes and disinfected the compartment. Nonimmune soldiers were then placed in each compartment, where they lived for several days. Neither soldier became ill, proving that the critical link in becoming infected was the mosquito.[16]

Private John R. Kissinger, one of the first enlisted men to volunteer for the experiment, was the first subject to come down with yellow fever after being exposed to the mosquitoes in Reed's spe-

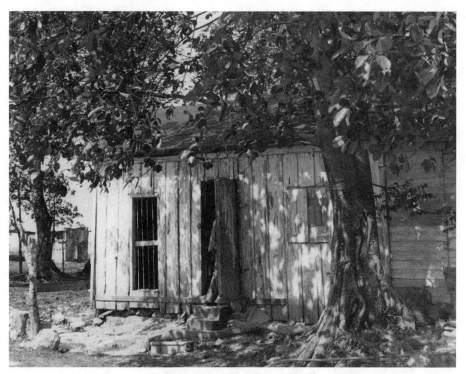

Building No. 1, Camp Lazear.

cially built compartment. On December 9, 1900, the day after Kissinger's diagnosis, Reed wrote to his wife to give her the "good" news. "As he had been in our camp for fifteen days before being inoculated and had had no other possible exposure, the case is as clear as the sun at noon-day, and sustains brilliantly and conclusively our conclusions," he wrote. "Tomorrow after we will have the Havana Board of Experts, Drs. Guiteras, Albertini, and Finlay, come out and diagnosis the case. I shan't tell them how the infection was acquired until after they have satisfied themselves concerning the character of the case, then I will let them know. I suppose old Dr. Finlay will be delighted beyond bounds, as he will see his theory at last fully vindicated." Later that night, Reed wrote a postscript to his letter: "Since writing the above [Kissinger] has been doing well. His temperature, which was 102.5 degrees at noon, has fallen to 101 degrees and his severe headache and backache have subsided considerably. Everything points, as far as it can at this stage, to a favorable termination for which I feel so happy."[17]

In all, the board's experiments produced eighteen cases of yellow fever, with Hospital Corps Private Charles G. Sonntag, who was bitten on February 7 and diagnosed with yellow fever on February 10, the last case of the disease to be produced at Camp Lazear. The day before Private Sonntag was bitten, Reed presented his second paper on the subject of yellow fever to the Pan-American Medical Congress in Havana. Titled "The Etiology of Yellow Fever— An Additional Note," it described the experiments at Camp Lazear and summarized the yellow fever board's findings:

- The mosquito *C. fasciatus* [later changed to *Stegomyia* and then later to *Aedes aegypti*, the name used today] was identified as the host for yellow fever.

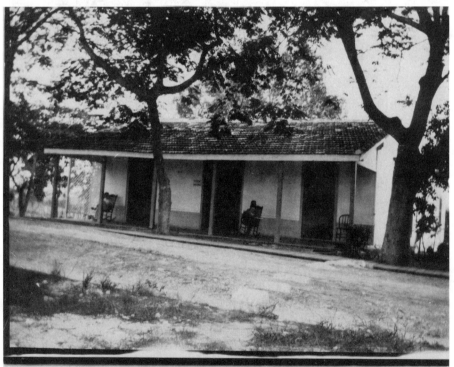

Building No. 2, used for yellow fever patients.

- Yellow fever is transmitted to humans by means of the bite of a mosquito that has previously fed on the blood of a diseased human.
- An incubation period of about twelve days is necessary after contamination in order for the mosquito to carry the infection.
- Humans bitten by the mosquito during the incubation period do not receive immunity to the disease.
- Yellow fever can be experimentally produced using blood taken from patients during the first and second days of the disease.
- Yellow fever is not conveyed by fomites, making disinfection of clothing and bedding unnecessary to prevent the spread of the disease.
- The only way a house can be infected is if it contains contaminated mosquitoes capable of passing along the disease.
- The spread of yellow fever can be most effectively controlled by destroying mosquitoes and protecting diseased patients from the bites of the insects.
- While the transmission of the disease has been identified, its specific cause remains a mystery. (It would be decades before the discovery of the electron microscope would allow researchers to actually view the living virus.)

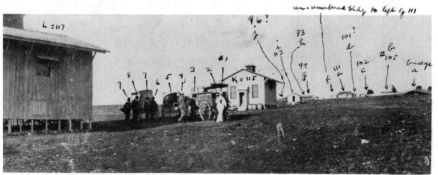

Yellow fever huts, Camp Columbia Post Hospital, Cuba.

Three days after delivering the speech in Havana, Reed sailed home, thus concluding the work of the US Army Yellow Fever Board. Back in the States, Reed resumed his duties as the curator of the Army Medical Museum and professor of bacteriology at the Army Medical School. Soon he was followed to Washington by Carroll, leaving Aristides Agramonte behind in Havana.

Once he was settled into his new routine, Reed wrote a revealing letter to his sister, Laura Reed Blincoe, that confessed that he was the only nonimmune member of the board who did not allow himself to be bitten by infected mosquitoes. "You know, or probably do not, that an order, early last June, sent me right down into the midst of yellow fever at Havana," he wrote. "Indeed I was sent down for the sole purpose of studying the disease. Dr. Lazear, of Baltimore, and Dr. Carroll, my assistant here, went with me. Both contracted the disease, and my dear friend Lazear, died of that disease! As for myself, I suppose that I was hardly worth killing and so escaped, although coming into the most intimate daily contact, *but I never permitted a mosquito to bite me!*"[18]

Upon his return to the States, Reed was a much-sought-after speaker, but he never received any compensation for his work, other than his regular army pay. For the most part, he sat on the sidelines, working as a teacher, while his research took on a life all its own. Two months after he arrived back in the States, Surgeon General Sternberg delivered a speech, without notes, to the Social Science Association in which he debunked the long-believed theory that yellow fever was contagious, capable of being passed by human contact. The *Washington Post* reporter who covered the speech described Sternberg as "perhaps the highest living authority on yellow fever. For more than a quarter of a century he has made it a study, and to that task he has brought not only special equipment as a microscopist [sic] and bacteriologist, but the keen, original intelligence so indispensable to any useful exploitation of that equipment. . . . Dr. Sternberg has rendered inestimable service to the cause of common sense and civilization."[19]

In September 1901, Reed went to Buffalo, New York, to present a paper on the prevention of yellow fever. He was about to deliver his address when President William McKinley was shot by an assassin elsewhere in the city, hardly an auspicious stimulus for an enlightened discussion of yellow fever. To make matters worse, Reed had been led to believe that his appearance was a congratulatory affair, but in reality it was little more than a platform from which his critics attempted to debunk his research.

One of his critics, Dr. A. N. Bell, Reed's former teacher at the Brooklyn City Hospital, attacked his former pupil for not acknowledging the role that unsterilized material played in the transmission of yellow fever. Eugene Wasdin argued that, while the disease could be transmitted by mosquitoes, it was not the only way. Reed offered an energetic rebuttal, but it must have pained him to be put in that position.

From that point on, Reed spent more time with his family, apparently giving up the hopes he had held for many years of advancing his career within the system. His ambition to become surgeon general seemingly evaporated overnight. In the year and a half after his return to the States, those who knew him felt that he was slowing down and often looked so tired that even walking seemed a chore.

On the evening of November 12, 1902, Reed was scheduled to deliver a lecture at the medical school, but he canceled, saying that he had eaten something at lunch that did not agree with him. The following day, he stayed in bed until noon and then went to work, only to be sent home by the hospital commander, Major William C. Borden. Together, they agreed that his symptoms indicated that he had appendicitis. Not feeling that it was an emergency, Borden made plans to operate the following week. Over the weekend, Reed seemed to show improvement, even to the point of requesting his usual breakfast.

As planned, Major Borden showed up at Reed's house on Monday morning and took him to the Army Hospital Barracks to be prepped for surgery. Before Reed was taken into the operating room, his old friend Major J. R. Kean arrived and had a conversation with him during which Reed, aware of the severity of his condition, said that he regretted that he had so little to leave to his family.

"It was difficult surgery," wrote Charles Morrow Wilson. "The appendix was hard to find. When the surgeon did locate it, he discovered that it was filled with pus and at one point perforated. Dr. Borden did his best. He litigated the appendix stump, inserted a gauze drainage, and packed it carefully. Reed reacted badly. For eighteen hours he suffered intense nausea. When the worst pain was abated he remained unusually nervous and depressed."

After the surgery, Major Kean called on him every day. Reed seemed obsessed with thoughts that he would leave his family with nothing in the way of a future. In an effort to boost his spirits, Kean told him that he had heard that Reed was going to be promoted to the rank of colonel, but Reed said he no longer cared about such things. Five days after the surgery, symptoms of peritonitis appeared, causing Reed to sink rapidly. He died on November 22, and he was buried at St. Thomas Church in Washington on a rainy day. His wife, Emilee, never visited him while he was in the hospital, and she was conspicuously absent at his funeral, setting off questions about whether she was in a doctor's care for emotional problems or simply felt estranged from her husband.

After his death, he was eulogized in numerous memorial services held by professional organizations, such as the New York Academy of Medicine and the University of Virginia. Within a year, the Walter Reed Memorial Association was established to raise money for Reed's family and to help pay for a suitable memorial. The goal was to raise $25,000, but it took more than four years to reach that amount. Contributors included Alexander Graham Bell, Surgeon General Sternberg, James Carroll, Carlos Finlay, William Gorgas, and members of the Rockefeller and

Morgan families. Construction of the memorial was delayed until the deaths of his wife and daughter so that their pensions would not be diminished by the added expenditure, but, not long after his death, Congress authorized funds for the construction of a general hospital for the army, and it was named for Walter Reed.

*   *   *

There were only twelve cases of yellow fever in Havana in January and February 1901, but those were traditionally low months for the disease. With the yellow fever board disbanded, William Gorgas, as Havana's chief sanitary officer, went about the business of ridding the city of the dreaded mosquito. It was undoubtedly one of the dirtiest cities in the world. Filth lay uncollected in the streets. Flies and mosquitoes filled the air. Sick people lay comatose on the streets from a variety of diseases, including yellow fever, typhoid, and dysentery. Gorgas took a methodical approach to the city's cleanup: he ordered the trash picked up and the sick segregated, and he used government money to build new roofs and install plumbing. He was so effective in his cleanup that Havana became an inviting showplace that attracted tens of thousands of Spanish immigrants, most without any source of income.

With the cleanup of the city proceeding smoothly, Gorgas turned his attention to eradicating yellow fever. He ordered that all patients with high fever had to be housed in a screened facility to prevent patients from coming into contact with mosquitoes. He used sulfur, formaldehyde, and insect powder to fumigate buildings containing mosquitoes. And, last but not least, he ordered the removal of any outdoor containers that could hold water and be used as a breeding ground for mosquitoes. Perhaps because he was not invited to participate in the experiments at Camp Lazear, Gorgas remained unconvinced that the mosquito was the *only* means by which yellow fever could be transmitted, and he ordered that buildings and clothing should continue to be disinfected.

That February, as he put his cleanup campaign into high gear, Gorgas authorized a Cuban physician, Dr. Juan Guiteras, to expand Reed's experiments in an effort to develop an immunization for yellow fever. It was during the early days of Guiteras's startup that Gorgas noted with humorous regret the passing of the last mosquito hatched by Walter Reed for his experiments.

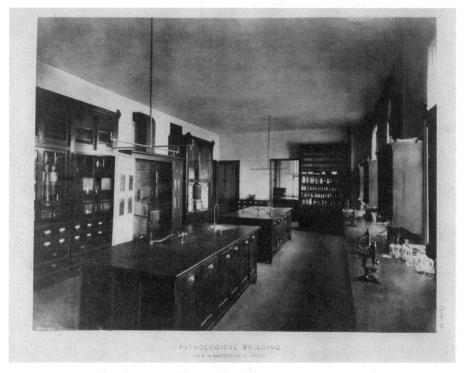

PATHOLOGICAL BUILDING
VIEW IN BACTERIOLOGICAL ROOM.

Bacteriological room in the pathological building, Cuba.

Gorgas told the *Times of Cuba*:

> The old lady was a veteran in every sense. She had given several persons yellow fever, but her greatest claim to celebrity was the fact that it had been fifty-seven days before the first case of fever and the last which she had given. . . . Dr. Guiteras had charge of the vaccination work and of the laboratory where the mosquitoes for this work were being bred. Our lady mosquito was,

therefore, directly under his care. She had given so many people yellow fever and was, therefore, so valuable for our prospective work, that we all, when at the hospital, would drop in to see how she was getting on and to pay our respects.

One morning about daylight I got a message stating that her ladyship was in a most critical and desperate plight, as some time during the night she had got her wing caught in a mesh of the mosquito netting and had struggled to free herself for so long a time that when she was discovered by the attendant in the morning she was almost dead. I rapidly dressed and hurried to the hospital. . . .

Two or three of the doctors on the staff of the hospital had been promptly called in and the services of several of our trained nurses had been likewise obtained. Her wing had been gently liberated from the mesh of the netting and her ladyship laid upon a soft bed of cotton batting. The oil stove was started up and the room brought to a very hot summer temperature, but it was all of no avail. She finally ceased to kick about 9 o'clock in the morning, and died with a larger attendance of doctors and nurses around her table than had ever been present of any mere human in the city of Havana.[20]

Impressed with the manner in which Walter Reed had been able to produce so many mild cases of yellow fever without any deaths, Guiteras sought to duplicate those experiments in order to determine whether a vaccine could be developed that would provide immunity by creating a case of the disease so mild as not to be harmful to the patient. Working out of the Las Animas Hospital in Havana, he recruited volunteers for his experiments. One of the first was a twenty-five-year-old nurse from New Jersey named Clara Maass. After being bitten several times in March, May, and June 1901 without results, she received a mosquito bite on August 14 that led to her death. Of eight cases produced by mosquitoes, three ended in death. Guiteras was both devastated and perplexed. How had Reed conducted his experiments without a single death? It would be a long time before Guiteras would understand that mosquitoes carry varying levels of the disease. The "lady" mosquito that Gorgas and others had laid to rest carried a strain of the disease that was less virulent than the strain that Guiteras's mosquitoes carried.

In the wake of Guiteras's experiments, James Carroll asked for permission to return to Cuba and carry on the research begun by the yellow fever board. On August 15, 1901, the adjutant general cabled Gorgas instructions to add Carroll's research to his budget and to pay the physician a per diem rate. Carroll arrived one week before Maass died. Of primary interest to him was whether yellow fever was filterable, as German researchers had proved to be the case with hoof and mouth disease in cattle. To investigate that possibility, he borrowed a number of infected mosquitoes from Guiteras and proceeded to vaccinate his first volunteer with yellow fever.

Once the diagnosis was made, Carroll drew blood from the patient on the third day of the illness, and it was allowed to stand and clot, providing material that could then be injected under the skin of another volunteer. It took only five days for the second volunteer to develop a mild case of the disease. At that point, Carroll heated some of the blood drawn from the first volunteer and injected it under the skin of three new volunteers, the result being that all three volunteers remained healthy past the safe point of ten days. Carroll felt that his experiment proved that the active agent in yellow fever was a living organism that could be controlled or destroyed by heat.

What Carroll did not realize was that his experiment had demonstrated that a living organism—in this case, the still-undiscovered yellow fever virus—could be transmitted from human to human. Shortly after Carroll completed the experiment, the army ordered the cessation of all experiments with human subjects, primarily because the death of nurse Maass had created a public outcry about the use of humans as experimental research subjects. The army had enough problems without being charged by the public with conducting Frankenstein-like experiments on God's creations.

*   *   *

As the 1900s exploded on the American consciousness, Panama seemed a distant footnote in world history. An S-shaped isthmus located between Costa Rica and Colombia, Panama has a land area equal to that of South Carolina. The isthmus was used for centuries as a thoroughfare by Indians traveling north and south, but it was not visited by white explorers until 1513, when Vasco Nunez de Balboa landed on the east coast and traveled through the swamps to the west coast, thus becoming the first white person ever to view the Pacific Ocean.

Americans first visited Panama in large numbers during the California gold rush of 1849. Easterners wishing to join the gold rush had three choices: they could make the overland trip and contend with hostile Indians, unpredictable weather, and towering mountain ranges; they could sail around the Horn, a distance of about fourteen thousand miles; or they could sail to Panama and cross the isthmus by wagon and then set sail for California by way of the Pacific Ocean. Thousands of Americans chose the Panama alternative, thus incorporating that country into still-evolving American history, especially with the completion of the Panama Railroad in 1855, an engineering feat that made Panama an important player in world trade.

Not until the Spanish-American War did the American military see the need for an east-west canal that would allow them to move warships from the Atlantic to the Pacific. By that time, Panama had become a province of Columbia, which had one of the strongest central governments in the region. The French had attempted to build a sea-level canal in the 1880s, but the project ended in failure, leaving the rights to a canal in the hands of a private French company. At first President William McKinley favored Nicaragua over Panama for the site of a canal, since it was explained to him that going through Nicaragua would be less expensive, but when the French company that owned the rights to a canal in Panama offered to sell those rights for $40 million, the commission studying the two plans voted in favor of Panama. Unfortunately, the Colombian government refused to allow the sale to take place.

After McKinley's death, which elevated Vice President Theodore Roosevelt to the office of the president, the United States concocted a plot with several prominent Panamanian families to separate Panama from Columbia. A few days before the plan was put into effect, Roosevelt sent the *USS Nashville* to Panama so that it would be there to block Columbian intervention in the revolt. Immediately after the revolt took place, the United States recognized Panama as an independent country, and the US Senate ratified a treaty in December 1903 that provided the United States exclusive control of a canal zone that was ten miles wide. The United States paid the Republic of Panama $10 million for the land strip and eventually agreed to pay the Panamanian government an additional $430,000 per year for use of the land.[21]

The actual building of the canal presented the US Army Corps of Engineers with a unique set of problems. Somehow they had to figure out how to maintain water levels on either side of the various locks needed to open up the canal to travel. And they had to figure out a way to deal with the biggest problem by far: the threat posed by mosquitoes for tropical diseases such as yellow fever and malaria. One report described the canal zone as "one of the hottest, wettest and most feverish regions in existence."

Interest in the construction of a canal coincided with Will Gorgas's departure from Havana in late 1902. In fact, before leaving Cuba, Gorgas wrote Surgeon General Sternberg a letter in which he suggested that the techniques used in Havana to rid the city of mosquitoes could be used in Panama to assist in the proposed canal project. Gorgas initially was recalled to Washington, but he was soon dispatched on official business to Paris, Suez, and Egypt, after which he was sent to Panama for an exploratory visit.

In January 1904, a seven-member Isthmian Canal Commission was organized. When it was learned that there were no physicians on the board, Roosevelt came under pressure from the American Medical Association and the news media to include a physician on the commission, if for no other reason than to offer expert guidance on the main obstacle to building the canal— yellow fever and malaria.

Roosevelt refused to install a physician on the commission, but he did see to it that William Gorgas, the individual who had the highest profile, other than the late Walter Reed, on the subject of mosquitoes was appointed to the post of chief sanitary officer of the Panama Canal Zone. Roosevelt's motivation is not difficult to understand. Mosquitoes were a highly charged issue at the turn of the century, and Roosevelt felt he would have more control of the issue if the "expert" was receiving a paycheck from the US Army.

Gorgas arrived in Panama on June 5, 1905, aboard the *SS Allianca*. With him was a party of eight—a chief sanitary engineer, a head nurse, Dr. Henry R. Carter, naval physician John Ross, Major James Turtle of the US Army, and two additional physicians. With no equipment to speak of, their mission was to rid the isthmus of mosquitoes and provide workmen with a safe environment.

Gorgas promptly asked the canal commission for workmen, and, just as promptly, the commission denied his request. Weren't eight experts enough to control the lowly mosquito? Frustrated by the commission's response, Gorgas cabled his superiors in Washington, only to be told that he should make all future requests by mail, considering the expense of cablegrams. Seemingly, the cap on Gorgas's frustrations was a statement by General George Davis, the first governor of the canal zone, that "a dollar spent on sanitation is like throwing it into the Bay."[22] As time went by, it became apparent to Gorgas that, while the commission was stingy with money for sanitation, it was quite generous in its funding for coffins. Gorgas also thought it odd that none of the commission members showed any interest in ever visiting Panama.

Gorgas did the best he could with what he had to work with. By November yellow fever was in full bloom in Panama. The news back home was filled with nightmarish stories of workers and visitors to the work site who were stricken by the disease. An architect who refused to authorize money for wire screening was one of the first to die, followed by office workers in the administration buildings and sailors who unloaded supplies from the ships. The American news media picked up on the story, and panic soon spread across the American political environment, as congressmen expressed fears that the project would never be completed.

The panic worked to Gorgas's advantage. Soon the supplies and additional personnel he requested were approved for delivery. Gorgas was very methodical in his attack on the mosquitoes. He got rid of the open rain barrels and troughs that Panamanians used to collect drinking water, and he ordered that oil be spread over any water collections that could not be drained. He also suggested that water should be transported from building to building through a system of pipes.

However, as Gorgas worked to remove the breeding grounds of the mosquitoes, the disease continued to find victims. Dr. Henry Carter told the story of a nurse who quietly slipped out of her quarters to join a young physician on a trip to Panama City, a hotspot of yellow fever activity. When the nurse came down with the disease, Carter rushed to her bedside: "I found her with yellow fever tossing from one side of the bed to the other. . . . Neither morphine nor cocaine quieted her. Finally I said, 'Child, you have a fine constitution and you ought to get well. But if you don't lie still in that bed you are going to die.' She insisted that she couldn't keep still, but suggested if Major [name deleted] would hold her hand she would try. I gave [the young doctor] a call and stationed him at his post. She quieted down immediately and the major sat by her all night. The girl got well, and it wasn't long after when I got cards to their wedding."[23]

Despite Gorgas's best efforts, the commission continued to label his mission in Panama a failure. It was not until Dr. Charles Reed, a former president of the American Medical Association, went to Panama on a fact-finding mission that the situation changed. Reed noted that yellow fever was being beaten, and he approved of Gorgas's methods. When he returned to the States, he attacked the commissioners as bunglers. The criticism that had the most resonance with the public was his report that the commission was paying $6.76 for a thirty-cent baby-bottle nipple. Armed with that news, President Roosevelt promptly fired all seven members of the commission.

Unfortunately, the new chairman, a railroad promoter who did not believe that mosquitoes could transmit yellow fever, recommended to the secretary of war that Gorgas should be fired and replaced with a man of more practical sensibilities. The secretary of war approved the recommendation and passed it along for the president's approval.

Not only did Roosevelt refuse to fire Gorgas, but also he ordered the new chairman to support Gorgas's efforts. It was at that point that Roosevelt did what no president before him had ever done—he left the United States and went to Panama to see for himself what was happening in that country. Roosevelt spent a great deal of time with Gorgas, and—impressed by what he saw—he saw to it that Gorgas was put in charge of an independent department and appointed to the commission.

By the time the canal was finished and opened to traffic in 1914, yellow fever had been completely eliminated. The death rate in the canal zone was six per thousand people, which was less than half the United States' rate of 14.1 per thousand. The healthiest state in America was still behind the canal zone in overall death rates. It was Gorgas, of course, who received credit for that success. He returned to the United States in triumph and was quickly elected president of the American Medical Association.

Over the next few years, Gorgas's star brightened even further.

In 1918, when the Rockefeller Foundation formed the Yellow Fever Commission, it chose Gorgas as director. The commission's first mission was to evaluate a yellow fever epidemic in Guayaquil, Ecuador. A Japanese-born scientist named Hideyo Noguchi, who had received worldwide attention for locating the syphilis spirochete in the brains of those already demented by the disease, was sent to Ecuador try to find the cause of yellow fever. Not long after he arrived, he identified a spirochete in the blood of six of twenty-seven patients, a discovery that prompted the commission to declare that Noguchi had solved the mystery. In 1920, Gorgas was coauthor of a paper that optimistically proclaimed: "The brilliant work of Noguchi in discovering the organism causing yellow fever already is having some effect on the control of the disease."[24]

No sooner did the commission celebrate Noguchi's "discovery" than there was word of a yellow fever epidemic in the West Coast of Africa. The Rockefeller Foundation responded by sending the Yellow Fever Commission to Africa, led by Gorgas. Unfortunately, Gorgas became ill before he arrived in Africa and was taken to London, where he was admitted to a military hospital at Willbank. The next day, he called for his wife and told her that he had suffered a stroke.

The British physicians predicted an early recovery, but Gorgas knew that he was dying. He had been in the hospital only briefly when the king of England stopped by to visit him. The king praised him for his work in Cuba and Panama and presented him with the Knight Commander of the Most Distinguished Order of St. Michael and St. George, saying, "I very sincerely appreciate the great work which you have done for humanity—work in which I take the greatest interest." Four weeks later, Gorgas died at the age of sixty-six. His body was returned to the United States, where he was buried with ceremony at Arlington.

*   *   *

Although Noguchi's theory about a yellow fever spirochete proved to be false, it did provide others with a starting point to locate the true cause of the disease. It was not until the yellow fever virus was viewable in an electron microscope that American scientist Wilbur Sawyer was able to develop the first successful vaccine against the disease in 1930. Dr. Max Theiler, a South African scientist, subsequently adapted the vaccine for mass production, an accomplishment for which he was awarded the 1951 Nobel Prize for medicine.

Thanks to the work of Carlos Finlay, who first advanced the idea that the mosquito was the carrier of the disease; Walter Reed and the other members of the first yellow fever board—James Carroll, Aristides Agramonte, and Jesse Lazear—who discovered the vital link as to how the disease was transmitted; William Gorgas, who developed the techniques by which mosquitoes could be eradicated; Drs. Sawyer and Theiler, for their work on developing a vaccine; and the availability of window and door screens and, later, air conditioning, yellow fever was eliminated as a major threat to the American continent, with the last epidemics occurring in 1905.

Even so, the yellow fever virus lingered in Central and South America for one hundred years, thriving in the mosquito-infested rainforests, a dark cloud of death hovering on America's distant horizon.

CHAPTER SIX

weapons of
mass destruction

Americans were first introduced to the concept of using disease as a weapon in 1763, when Lord Jeffrey Amherst, a general who was in charge of all British forces in North America, ordered that blankets used in a smallpox hospital be given to Native Americans in an effort to infect them with the disease.

"You will do well to try to inoculate the Indians by means of blankets, as well as to try every other method that can serve to extirpate the execrable race," Amherst wrote in a letter to a subordinate officer. Replied the officer, who was stationed in Philadelphia: "We gave them two blankets and an handkerchief out of the smallpox hospital. I hope it will have the desired effect." History records that it did have the "desired" effect and resulted in an epidemic among the Delaware and Shawnee Indians, who were especially vulnerable to the disease, since it was new to North America, and they had built up no natural immunities.

Amherst's war crimes against the Indians allowed him to defeat his real enemies, the French, thus making it possible for him to acquire Canada for England. It was to pay tribute to the man, later to be known as Lord Amherst, that the Massachusetts city was named in his honor. Lord Amherst was "the most glamorous military hero in the New World," notes historian Frank

Prentice Rand. "The name was so obvious in 1759 as to be almost inevitable."[1]

Except for the episode with the blankets—Native American histories charged that the practice continued well into the 1800s, but no documentary evidence of that, other than oral histories, has yet surfaced—there were instances when smallpox was used in a less overt way, such as in 1862 when white medical authorities in British Columbia reportedly vaccinated whites but refused to vaccinate Indians during an epidemic that wiped out half the Indian population from Victoria to Alaska.

Biological warfare faded into the background until the early 1900s, when Germany expanded the concept of biological warfare through the use of chemical weapons designed to cause mass casualties. The first chemical attack involved chlorine gas that was used against French and Algerian troops on April 22, 1915, at the Belgium city of Ypres. "Suddenly . . . three flares rose from an observation balloon over the German lines and burst against the darkening eastern sky," wrote Charles E. Heller of the Combat Studies Institute, US Army Command. He continued:

> German artillery commenced a fierce bombardment that landed to the rear of the French and British lines in the Ypres sector. Then . . . an eerie silence fell over the area. Peering across the battle field, men of two French divisions, the 87th Territorial and the 45th Algerian, saw blue-white wisps of haze rising from the German trenches. The haze swirled about, gathered in a cloud that slowly turned yellow-green and began to drift across the terrain at a height of up to six feet.
>
> As the cloud drifted, it settled into every depression in the landscape. Finally, the gentle northeasterly wind brought it spilling into the French trenches, silently enveloping the occupants in a misty, deadly embrace. To the north and southwest of the now mist-enshrouded French positions, British and Canadian troops looked into the haze and, to their amazement, saw soldiers, many without weapons, emerge from the cloud, "running wildly, and in confusion" toward positions to the rear.

Terror-stricken Algerians ran by the startled Dominion troops, coughing and clutching their throats. Moments later French soldiers staggered by, "blinded, coughing, chests heaving, faces an ugly purple color, lips speechless with agony."[2]

The gas killed all those who breathed it, filling the soldiers' lungs with fluids that suffocated them within a matter of minutes as attacking German soldiers, wearing masks made of hemp and soaked in baking soda, overran the French and Algerian lines. A month later, the Germans released 264 tons of chlorine gas along a twelve-kilometer line southeast of Warsaw, Poland. Before the war ended, more than two hundred chemical attacks were documented, the largest taking place at Rhiems, where 550 tons of chlorine gas was released by the Germans. By the conclusion of the war, the German gases had produced an estimated 1.3 million casualties.[3]

The German gas attacks created a delicate political situation for the United States. At The Hague Conference of 1899, the agenda item prohibiting the use of shells filled with asphyxiating gas passed with only one dissenting vote. The American representative, naval Capt. Alfred Mahan, voted against the ban, declaring that "it was illogical and not demonstrably humane to be tender about asphyxiating men with gas, when all were prepared to admit that it was allowable to blow the bottom out of an ironclad at midnight, throwing four or five hundred men into the sea, to be choked by water, with scarcely the remotest chance of escape."[4] Secretary of State John Hay had instructed Mahan to vote against the ban because he did not think it made sense to limit the types of weapons that the American military might need in future wars.

Once World War I broke out in Europe, it became increasingly obvious that the United States would be drawn into the conflict, despite President Woodrow Wilson's attempts to maintain strict neutrality. Meanwhile, America's refusal to ban the use of chemical warfare at The Hague created public relations problems. The

Allies depicted the gas attacks as cruel and inhumane in an effort to influence American public opinion, but the Wilson administration was hard pressed to repudiate the position that America took at The Hague. Was chemical warfare permissible, as Mahan had argued, or did it cross the bounds of civilized standards of warfare? The Wilson administration grappled with that dilemma until the Allies retaliated against the Germans with similar weapons, thus moving closer to the American position.

Ironically, when the United States declared war on Germany on April 6, 1917, the American military was totally unprepared for chemical warfare. Not only were there no American experts who had knowledge of offensive chemical warfare, there was no plan in place to develop and manufacture gas masks that could be used to protect American soldiers. America agreed to send the Allies a division of soldiers right away, but military planners estimated that they would be engaged in combat for several months before they could be equipped with defensive gas equipment.

The peace treaties that followed the end of World War I, including the Treaty of Berlin—a separate treaty between the United States and Germany—prohibited the importation or manufacture by Germany of poisonous gases or liquids. In 1925 the United States signed the Geneva Protocol, which stated: "Whereas the use in war of asphyxiating, poisonous or other gases, and all analogous liquids, materials or devices, has been justly condemned by the general opinion of the civilized world; and whereas the prohibition of such use has been declared in Treaties to which the majority of the Powers of the World are Parties; and to the end that this prohibition shall be universally accepted as a part of International Law, binding alike the conscience and the practice of nations; declare: that the High Contracting Parties, so far as they are not already Parties to Treaties prohibiting such use, accept this prohibition, agree to extend this prohibition to the use of bacteriological methods of warfare and agree to be bound as between themselves according to the terms of this declaration."

The Geneva Protocol of 1925 was observed by the international community until the early 1930s, when the Imperial Japanese Army began a massive secret program to develop biological weapons of mass destruction. Once America became aware of Japan's goals, it took the threat seriously and set up an intelligence network to monitor that country's progress. The Japanese evidently felt that chemical weapons, which worked so well in the flatlands of Europe, were unsuited for the jungle and mountainous terrain in which it expected to wage future wars. What the Japanese military wanted were infectious diseases that could be weaponized and used under a variety of conditions.

By 1939, it became obvious to American investigators that Japan's weapon of choice was a disease that had created the largest and most frightening epidemics in American history— yellow fever![5]

*   *   *

The peace treaties that emerged from World War I were not so much guarantees of peace as they were expressions of an armed truce. For simplicity's sake, many historians date the start of World War II as September 1, 1939, when Germany invaded Poland, but Japan's invasion of China and its occupation of Manchuria in 1931 and 1932 are sometimes used as the true starting date. Up until that time, the world had remained essentially at peace because it was believed that the League of Nations would mobilize public opinion against any nation that crossed international boundaries for the purpose of initiating preemptive strikes against perceived enemies.

Once Japan challenged the League of Nations' authority—and proved it to be a weak, ineffectual organization whose bark was worse than its bite—it opened the door for other nations to use military means to pursue foreign policy objectives. Three years later, Italian dictator Benito Mussolini put the Japanese challenge to a test by invading Ethiopia. As it had done with Japan, the League of Nations took no action against Italy. The Ethopia conquest was followed by the joint decision of Mussolini and German's new chancellor, Adolf Hitler, to assist in the overthrow of the Spanish Republic for the purpose of installing a Fascist dictatorship. Again, the League of Nations debated the issue among its members, but took no action.

By early 1939, it was clear to Hitler that there was no organized force to stop his Nazi Party from pursuing its nationalist goals of uniting Germany with Austria, Poland, and Czechoslovakia. Hitler's seizure of Austria and Czechoslovakia by the end of March 1939—and his publicly stated goals of acquiring Poland—convinced Great Britain and France that Hitler's real mission was the control of eastern Europe.

The first seven months of World War II were lopsided in Germany's favor. Hitler had built a powerful military machine, which, though smaller than the combined armies of Great Britain and France, was better trained. The German *blitzkrieg*, as it later was called, rolled over French and British defenders with frightening efficiency. The French surrendered in June 1940, leaving Great Britain to face the German military machine with no allies and little prospect of success.

Great Britain desperately wanted the United States to enter the war, but President Franklin Roosevelt did not feel that public sentiment would support America's entry into it. Under the American system of government, only Congress can make a declaration of war—and at that time Congress was not being pressured by voters back home to take decisive action. All that changed, of course, on December 7, 1941, when Japan sent one hundred fighting planes, torpedo bombers, and dive bombers, along with a fleet of midget submarines, to attack the American naval base at Pearl Harbor, Hawaii. More than 2,300 American sailors, soldiers, and marines were killed, with another 1,272 wounded and 960 missing.

The Japanese Foreign Ministry sent a coded message to its embassy in Washington, with orders that the message was to be decoded and typed in English and delivered to the White House at precisely 1 PM, twenty-five minutes before the attack was to begin. Unfortunately, the first secretary at the embassy could not find anyone with the needed security clearance to type the message, and he was forced to type it out himself. Because he was a slow typist, by the time he finished, the attack had already began, a mistake that prevented the White House from cabling an early warning to Pearl Harbor.

In the angry days that followed, President Roosevelt referred to the sneak attack as a day that would "live in infamy." Without the attack, it is questionable if the United States would have entered the war, but, because of it, Congress issued a declaration of war against both Japan and Germany.

One of the first things that the US military did after the attack on Pearl Harbor was to vaccinate all active-duty personnel against yellow fever. The fear was that Japan would launch a biological attack against the United States with the same efficiency and determination that it had displayed at Pearl Harbor. Suspected targets were California, the Midwest, and the South, along with all overseas areas where there was likely to be ground combat. At that time, all American military personnel already received typhoid, smallpox, and tetanus vaccines. Any soldiers who refused to take the vaccines were subject to a military court martial, a rule that was put into effect during World War I and remained on the books.

Considering the intelligence that the American military had gathered about Japan's research with yellow fever, the vaccine order made sense. There was only one problem: A safe vaccine would not be developed for mass production until after the war, which meant that the only yellow fever vaccine available was one that was not licensed for civilian use in the United States. The available vaccine contained human serum, and many of the vials used were contaminated with hepatitis B, a virus that often mimics the symptoms of yellow fever and leads to death or permanent liver damage.

Unfortunately, shortly after the vaccinations began, American soldiers experienced an epidemic of hepatitis B. More than 50,000 soldiers were hospitalized for treatment of hepatitis B, and subsequent investigation discovered that about 330,000 individuals had been infected by the vaccination.[6] Because of the epidemic, now known to be the largest hepatitis outbreak ever recorded, the yellow fever vaccinations were halted in April 1942. Follow-up studies reported that the soldiers fared better than expected, with no increase in deaths from chronic liver disease and only a slight increase in deaths from liver cancer. It was not illegal at that time for the military to use unlicensed vaccines, but clearly it had a chilling effect on the military's willingness to expose troops to additional untested ones.[7]

No sooner did the United States enter the war in Europe than it realized that it was going to face a new chemical war threat. Before the start of the war, Germany had instructed its scientists to develop a new substance superior to the old chlorine and mustard gases used during World War I. What they came up with were quick-kill nerve gases such as tabun and sarin, anticholinesterase agents that work by blocking the enzyme that the body uses to destroy used nerve transmitters. The effects are twofold: the individual is incapacitated, then the body poisons itself.

"The symptoms of nerve-gas poisoning are diverse and spectacular," says J. Perry Robinson, who wrote his thesis at Oxford University on certain aspects of chemical warfare. "In a comparatively inactive man an exposure to sarin of 15 mg-min/m dims the vision, the eyes hurt and become hard to focus. This may last for a week or more. At 40 mg-min/m, the chest feels tight, breathing is difficult, there is coughing, drooling at the mouth, nausea, heartburn, and a twitching of the muscles. At 55, there is a strangling tightness and aching of the chest, vomiting, cramps, tremors, and involuntary defecation and urination. At 70, severe convulsions will set in followed closely by collapse, paralysis, and death."[8]

Once details of the German nerve gases became known, the US Army quickly diverted its attention from yellow fever, a suspected but unproven threat, to focus on the more immediate threat posed by nerve gas. Gas masks were provided for civilians as well as soldiers. To discourage first use of nerve gas by Germany, President Roosevelt pledged massive retaliation against German cities if biological or chemical weapons were used against US soldiers or civilians. The United States, Great Britain, and the other Allied countries involved in the war manufactured poison gases in large quantities so that they would be prepared to fight back at the first sign of a chemical attack. It never came. For whatever reason, Germany declined to use its chemical arsenal, a decision that baffled some Allied military planners.

Meanwhile, Japan set up a top-secret biological warfare research center in China, where scientists conducted experiments on a variety of diseases, including yellow fever, bubonic plague, anthrax, and syphilis. There was no shortage of human subjects for the experiments at Unit 731. Thousands of prisoners of war from America, Great Britain, and China were herded through the facility and subjected to a series of nightmarish experiments in which they were injected with yellow fever, bubonic plague, and typhoid. In winter 1942, more than fifteen hundred American soldiers captured in the Philippines were given injections and accompanied to China by Japanese researchers. The American POWs who died during that first winter were stacked outside to freeze and then collected in the spring by surviving POWs, who were instructed to bury some bodies in a mass grave and to carry the remaining bodies to a building where they could be dissected.

American efforts to develop poison gases were led by George W. Merck, the president of a drug company that was a household name across America. Work got underway in 1943 at Camp Detrick, an army base in rural Maryland that was only a short distance from Washington, DC. The base was surrounded with machine-gun-toting guards, and the researchers were asked to keep handguns nearby. With little more than a shell in place, the secret base was quickly expanded to more than two hundred fifty buildings capable of housing five thousand personnel.

As soon as the facilities were equipped with the latest scientific tools for the exploration of killer diseases and poisonous gases, the Detrick scientists began work on developing a strain of anthrax that could be used to kill enemy troops. They also experimented with agricultural diseases that could be spread by aircraft over Japanese rice fields and German potato fields. A third area of focus was developing deadly toxins that could be sprayed directly on enemies, a pursuit that led to botulinum toxin, one of the most potent poisons known to man.

None of the weapons of mass destruction developed at Detrick were used in World War II. That is because a second research facility located at Los Alamos, New Mexico, was at work on a far superior weapon of mass destruction—the atomic bomb. The technology that allowed scientists to split the uranium atom was developed by two German scientists just prior to the start of World War II. They learned that, when the uranium was split by nuclear fission, it generated more than two hundred million electron volts of energy that could be channeled into a chain reaction of unimaginable force.

Aware of the horrific implications associated with atomic energy—and fearful that Germany would find a way to build an atomic bomb of its own—American scientists asked President Roosevelt in 1939 to establish a top-secret research project to study atomic-bomb development. In 1942, when it became apparent that the scientists had successfully sustained a nuclear chain reaction, the US War Department took over the project for the sole purpose of producing an atomic bomb.

The following year, the project was named the Manhattan Engineer District and turned over to army engineers for development. Once the engineers felt that they had collected enough nuclear materials to fuel an atomic bomb, the project was handed over to a specially built laboratory at Los Alamos, New Mexico, where a young American physicist named J. Robert Oppenheimer took charge of actually building and testing the bomb. The first artificial nuclear explosion in history took place on July 16, 1945, in a New Mexico desert near Alamogordo.

Three months earlier, President Franklin Roosevelt died, catapulting Vice President Harry S Truman into the presidency. One of the first shocks he encountered upon entering office was that the United States was developing an atomic bomb. Roosevelt had kept the project under such a tight veil of secrecy that not even the vice president was advised of its progress. Truman saw no reason to terminate the project and proceeded with the management of the war in Europe. Less than a month after he took office, Germany agreed to an unconditional surrender, thus allowing the new president to focus on winning the war against Japan.

Using the surrender of Germany as a wedge, Truman called on the Japanese to stop fighting in the Pacific and accept his terms of unconditional surrender. Without being specific, he promised the destruction of Japan if they refused to do so. When the Japanese expressed no interest in surrendering, Truman authorized an air strike against Hiroshima, a city of about 350,000 people. The bomb was delivered by the Enola Gay, a B-29 bomber outfitted to carry the four-ton bomb.

On August 6, 1945, the Enola Gay took off from a US air base in the western Pacific and flew six and a half hours to Hiroshima, where it dropped the bomb on the unsuspecting city. The resulting fireball reached a temperature of several million degrees centigrade and created a cloud that rose nearly twenty miles. People within a one-kilometer radius of the blast were instantly burned to death. Those who were within a three- to five-kilometer radius had their skin burned from their bodies. In all, the bomb killed more than 155,200 people, most of whom were women and children.

Truman then issued a second ultimatum to the Japanese, but they ignored it with the same silence that had greeted his first warning. Consequently, Truman ordered that a second atomic bomb be dropped on Nagasaki, a city of about two hundred thousand. This time, about seventy thousand Japanese civilians were killed outright, with many more destined to die of leukemia and other cancers. Two days later, Truman announced that many more atomic bombs would be dropped unless the Japanese surrendered immediately. The Japanese agreed to accept the same terms that had been offered to Germany, provided the emperor could retain his sovereignty. The Allies agreed, but only with the understanding that the emperor would submit to the authority of the Supreme Allied Commander in Japan, General Douglas MacArthur.

Japan's surrender was a great victory for the United States, one that saved the lives of thousands of American servicemen, but the victory was achieved at great cost in world public opinion. By becoming the first nation to use atomic bombs against civilians, the United States, which had tried to avoid war with both Germany and Japan, had become the world's leading authority on weapons of mass destruction.

With the surrender of Japan, the scientists at Unit 731 destroyed evidence of war crimes and returned to Japan, where MacArthur offered them protection against prosecution in exchange for their secret records and their help in translating them. Fearing that the Soviet Union, by then perceived to be the next threat to American security, would get its hands on information pirated out of Unit 731, the American military shifted its strategic planning from atomic weapons to biological weapons. Germ warfare was viewed as the perfect weapon, in that it could destroy people in large numbers without damaging buildings. The Japanese records from Unit 731 were invaluable because the Japanese had no qualms about experimenting with human subjects, something American researchers were forbidden to do.

Demoted to second-class status by the development of the atomic bomb, Camp Detrick got new life at the end of World War II. There was a lively debate within the military over the value of biological warfare—critics said it was too unpredictable and made Americans look like the bad guys; the knowledge obtained in Japan, they argued, should be used to cure disease, not inflict it on others—but the argument was won by those who maintained that the United States could best protect itself by developing a full range of weapons of mass destruction. Once again, Camp Detrick was designated the focal point of America's biological warfare research, with a second testing facility built on a small island off the coast of Mississippi.

In the years immediately following World War II, the world was filled with rumors of covert biological warfare. Newspaper articles accused Jews of causing a cholera outbreak in Egypt in 1947, and they accused the United States of testing biological weapons against Canada's Eskimo population in 1949, causing a deadly plague epidemic. Most people were horrified by talk of biological warfare, but there were others who welcomed it. In 1947 Australian microbiologist MacFarlane Burnet, who later won the Nobel Prize for medicine, recommended biological weapons as a means of combating world overpopulation. He told a government committee in 1948 that yellow fever would be the perfect population-control device for countries with appropriate mosquito vectors.[9]

No one understood the terror associated with yellow fever more than America because no country had ever been attacked by the disease with such catastrophic results. Once researchers at Camp Detrick had access to the results of the Japanese experiments, they went to work on finding means of weaponizing the disease. Scientists saw two possibilities: infecting mosquitoes with the disease, by the millions, so that they could be released on an unsuspecting population—or finding a way to spread the disease by means of an aerosol spray.

Thanks to the research of Dr. Wilbur Sawyer, who developed the yellow fever vaccine, they had guidelines for handling the infectious material during their research. In his report to the Rockefeller Foundation, which was written two years before he perfected a vaccine, Sawyer detailed the process he went through to handle the infectious material, stating six conclusions about the methods used:

- The yellow fever virus may be preserved for up to 154 days in the blood or liver tissue of infected monkeys if the material is dried in a vacuum while in the frozen state and kept in the refrigerator in sealed glass containers. A gradual diminution of virulence is noticeable in the older specimens.
- If infectious blood is dried in a vacuum at room temperature, instead of in the frozen state, and is stored in sealed containers in the refrigerator, the virus may survive as long as 155 days.
- The virus may be preserved for at least thirty days in liver kept continuously frozen.
- Storage of blood or liver in 50 percent glycerin in the refrigerator will usually keep the virus alive for sixty days and may do so for one hundred days, but, with the injection of the older material, there is a marked tendency toward lengthening of the incubation period and an increase in the number of recoveries.
- Yellow fever virus in citrated or clotted blood, when kept in the refrigerator, dies out rapidly.
- The most satisfactory method of preserving strains of the yellow fever virus in the laboratory consists of freezing and drying blood taken from a monkey on the first day of an attack of experimental yellow fever and storing the dry material in sealed glass tubes in a cold place.

Once scientists understood the virus's storage potential, they focused on a delivery system. Obviously, the best carrier was the mosquito itself. The army's yellow fever board had demonstrated nearly a half century earlier how mosquitoes could be infected with the disease, and the board had proved how mosquitoes could be harvested in large numbers in the laboratory. Camp Detrick, using its testing facility near Mississippi, proceeded to produce 100 million yellow fever mosquitoes each week for possible use against enemy troops. Where those mosquitoes were tested is not known. Between 1956 and 1958, there were reports that the US Army carried out field tests in Savannah, Georgia, and Avon Park, Florida, by releasing mosquitoes into residential neighborhoods. After each test, people became ill, with some of them dying, and they were monitored by army personnel disguised as public health officials who tested and photographed the victims. Army spokesmen denied that the mosquitoes were infected with yellow fever, but details of the experiments remain classified.

During the Korean War, the Soviet Union, China, and North Korea accused the United States of using biological warfare against North Korea and China, but an international panel of scientists who investigated the charges found no evidence that such weapons were being used.[10] The following year, several American journalists accused General MacArthur of using yellow fever mosquitoes against North Korea. The army denied the charges, and the journalists who published the allegations were charged with sedition, but none of them were ever convicted.

One of the scientists at Camp Detrick who worked on the yellow fever project was Bill Patrick, a young researcher who felt that viruses were the key to an effective weapons arsenal. He advanced quickly at Detrick and soon was put in charge of the facility's virus factories. He discovered that chicken eggs were the cheapest and most effective way of incubating yellow fever viruses.[11] Some of that work was farmed out to the Pine Bluff arsenal, which, at its peak, turned out a reported 120,000 yellow-fever-infected eggs a week. Little is known about the process by which Patrick was able to aerosol the disease, but, by the early 1960s, America had a formidable yellow fever arsenal that had the capability to wipe out entire countries.

Events in Central America in 1956 may have given military strategists pause about ever using such weapons on a large scale. On February 12, 1956, the *New York Times* ran a story under the headline: "Fever of the Jungle Marching North: Disease Approaching Mexico and British Honduras—Not Held by Natural Barrier." Dr. Fred Soper, director of the Pan American Sanitary Organization, was quoted as warning that yellow fever could reach Mexico within one year. A yellow fever epidemic in Mexico would create panic in the United States—and the army understood that better than anyone.

The epidemic never took place, but apparently it did influence the army's decision to put yellow fever on the back burner in order to focus on other viruses. Besides concern about unleashing an epidemic that could somehow affect the US mainland, the army had to contend with the danger associated with managing millions of infected mosquitoes. The testing facility off the coast of Mississippi was shut down, according to Bill Patrick, because "there were too many mosquitoes and other arthropods that could probably take up some of the diseases we were disseminating and spread them to our civilian population." For that reason, the facility was moved from Mississippi to the Utah desert, and then shut down again.[12]

Dr. Ned Hayes, a medical epidemiologist with the viral disease branch of the Centers for Disease Control, says he thinks the United States abandoned its yellow fever program because it proved to be inefficient as an aerosol weapon. "It is not a virus that is transmitted naturally by aerosol," he says. "There have been laboratory infections that presumably were due to aerosolizing of the virus, so if you are working with the virus in the laboratory, you have to be careful. You have to recognize that it can be transmitted in a laboratory setting. They did some experiments with monkeys and they were able to transmit the virus by aerosol, so it's not that it can't be used as an aerosol. My understanding is that it's just not stable enough to be effective."[13]

*   *   *

The Vietnam War, which went from a simmering conflict in the early 1960s to a major commitment of United States troops by the mid- to late 1960s, proved the disadvantages of biological weapons. Thick jungle canopies of the type that define most of Vietnam render biological weapons useless for tactical purposes. The US military gave a great deal of thought to infecting enemy populations with smallpox, a weapon that was favored by American biological warfare researchers, but some scientists felt that smallpox might prove difficult to control in that particular situation—and there was concern that it could be traced back to the United States, thus providing the potent American peace movement with headline-grabbing ammunition to demand the withdrawal of all troops from Vietnam.

One problem the military had during that time was managing public opinion. Since the troops in Vietnam were draftees from the heartland, where opposition to the war was growing with lightning speed, military planners had to consider the effects of negative publicity on their troops in the field. In 1968 noted journalist Seymour M. Hersh published a book titled *America's Hidden Arsenal*, which examined the military's capabilities for chemical and biological warfare. The book followed on the heels of several public efforts by some of the country's most prominent scientists who questioned the use of disease as a military tactic. And, of course, Camp Detrick, which changed its name to Fort Detrick, came under siege as antiwar protestors marched outside the barbed wire, spotlighting the military's most sensitive top-secret facility.

One of the most troublesome scientists of that era, at least for President Richard Nixon's administration, was Matthew Meselson, a Harvard biologist with top-secret clearances who was very much opposed to the use of biological weapons. He proposed a three-pronged public-health response to the threat of biological weapons: prevention, shielding, and treatment. During the height of the protests, Meselson had an airport encounter with his old Harvard colleague, Henry Kissinger, who had just been appointed Nixon's national security adviser. Kissinger was aware of Meselson's concerns about germ warfare and asked for advice on what should be done. Meselson responded with, "Let me think about it. I'll write you some papers."[14]

One of Meselson's studies, dated September 1969, argued that biological weapons, while extremely destructive, were unnecessary. Wrote the authors of *Germs: Biological Weapons and America's Secret War:* "A light aircraft could deliver enough to kill populations over several thousand square miles . . . but the disease could spread far beyond the target area or create a long-term epidemic hazard. The same fickleness was true of incapacitating germs. . . . In an attack they might actually cause a large number of deaths among both enemy personnel and intermingled civilians, or might cause too little incapacitation to be militarily effective. [Meselson] asserted that the nation's strategic nuclear forces were enough to deter attack. 'We have no need to rely on lethal germs weapons and would lose nothing by giving up the option,' he wrote. 'Our major interest is to keep other nations from acquiring them.'"

Two months later, in November 1969, Nixon shocked his right-wing supporters by announcing that he was shutting down America's offensive biological warfare program. "The U.S. shall renounce the use of lethal biological agents and weapons, and all other methods of biological warfare," Nixon said at a press conference at Fort Detrick. "The U.S. will confine its biological research to defensive measures."

Almost overnight, America began to play a leading role in the international movement to ban biological weapons. The initial reason America got into the germ warfare business—to protect overseas troops and the homeland against chemical and biological attacks—was overlooked by military strategists at the conclusion of World War II, who seemed to get caught up in the mindless inertia of developing an offensive arsenal second to none in the world. Once the Nixon administration understood that biological weapons were a greater threat to the United States than to any of the nation's enemies, it became obvious that their spread must be stopped. As a result, the United States, along with the Soviet Union and more than one hundred other nations, signed the Biological and Toxin Weapons Convention, which prohibited the possession of any biological toxins not needed for research to develop defensive vaccines and protective equipment needed to shield soldiers and civilians from a biological weapons attack.

However, the Nixon administration made a distinction between biological weapons and chemical weapons. In Vietnam, instead of dipping into its biological warfare arsenal, the US military used chemical weapons that were not specifically banned by the treaty. The most extensively used was a dioxin-powered herbicide called Agent Orange. The military's stated purpose for using Agent Orange was to defoliate the jungle canopy so that the air war could be conducted with greater efficiency, but the peace movement uncovered a far different motive.

M. F. Kahn, an investigator for the International War Crimes Tribunal, went to Vietnam for the purpose of assessing the use and effectiveness of Agent Orange. What he and his team members concluded "beyond doubt" was that "concentrated attacks on the food supplies of the Vietnamese people was the main target of the so-called defoliants in Vietnam. The obvious ineffectiveness of the chemicals on the declared target—the jungle—contrasts sharply with the relative efficiency against crops and food and trees."[15] Despite military assurances of Agent Orange's safety, thousands of Vietnam civilians were poisoned by the chemical (the Vietnam government put the number at 500,000), and thousands of American soldiers were exposed to the compound while in Vietnam and later suffered a variety of ill effects, including birth defects in their offspring. Agent Orange was not designed to target humans, but that was the effect it had in Vietnam, thus proving arguments made by scientists that chemical and biological weapons are almost impossible to control once unleashed.

Dr. Thomas W. McGovern, a former army major who was assigned to the Medical Research Institute of Infectious Diseases at Fort Detrick in the 1990s, long after the Nixon administration halted research on offensive biological weapons, is not convinced that fungal toxins such as trichothecene mycotoxins were not used in Southeast Asia between 1974 and 1981. "A total of 397 attacks delivered by means of aerosol, droplet clouds, aircraft rockets, bombs, canisters, handheld weapons, and booby traps resulted in more than 6,300 deaths in Laos, 981 deaths in Kampuchea and 3,042 deaths in Afghanistan," he has written. "In Laos, the attacks were described as yellow rain; a sticky yellow liquid fell and sounded like rain or looked like a yellow cloud of dust, powder, mist, smoke, or insect spray. The liquid dried rapidly to form a powder. Most attacks involved the use of yellow pigment, but some attacks involved red, green, white, or brown smoke or vapor. More than 80 percent of the attacks were delivered by means of air-to-surface rockets."[16]

The Nixon administration apparently lived up to the terms of the Biological and Toxin Weapons Convention of 1972, but it explored loopholes that allowed it to develop biological weapons that could be used for assassination purposes. After Nixon's resignation in the wake of the Watergate scandal, the US Senate held a series of hearings to investigate alleged wrongdoing in the intelligence community.

The Senate learned that the Central Intelligence Agency (CIA) had worked with researchers at Fort Detrick to plot a series of assassinations using exotic biological weapons. Targets included Patrice Lumumba, the elected prime minister of the Congo (the CIA wanted to kill him with botulism), and Cuban dictator Fidel Castro (the CIA hatched a plan to kill him with tuberculosis germs sprinkled on his deep-sea diving gear). Among the weapons found in the CIA arsenal were anthrax, tularemia, encephalitis, tuberculosis, lethal snake venom, and salmonella food poisoning.

*   *   *

With a few minor exceptions, biological weapons evaded public discussion for nearly twenty years. Not until the Persian Gulf War of 1991 to 1992 did the subject of biological weapons again make news headlines. When Iraq invaded Kuwait on August 2, 1990, to seize disputed land, the George Bush administration released intelligence reports that stated that Iraqi president Saddam Hussein's army had an arsenal that included biological weapons. The US government was not specific about the range of weapons in the possession of Iraq's army, but both anthrax and nerve gas were mentioned as possible threats. When the Bush administration made the decision to go to war with Iraq, the US military was unprepared for combat action against an enemy that possessed biological weapons. Anthrax vaccines were available to the military, but there was not a single soldier or reservist who had ever been inoculated against anthrax.

Researchers at Fort Detrick were asked to solve that problem—and quickly. Their solution was to either vaccinate each and every soldier or supply them with potent antibiotics that would be effective in treating the disease. Either "solution" was certain to kill an unknown percentage of soldiers because of side effects of the drugs and vaccinations.

Despite repeated warnings that Iraq's army planned to use biological or chemical weapons, no such use was ever confirmed.

However, in the months following the war, American soldiers began showing symptoms of biological or chemical poisoning. Since the American military denied the existence of such weapons on the battlefield by either side, no linkage was ever established. In time, the symptoms were given a name—the Gulf War Syndrome. Neither the affected soldiers nor the public ever believed government claims that biological and chemical weapons were not used in the war.

As the years went by after the Persian Gulf War, public concerns about biological and chemical weapons again waned, to the point of being nonexistent as George W. Bush was sworn in as president in 2001. All that changed on September 11, 2001, when Islamic terrorists flew two hijacked jetliners into both buildings of the World Trade Center, killing hundreds of innocent civilians. Within hours of the attack, US soldiers were on the ground with sensitive detectors to determine whether the terrorists had released deadly germs. None were found, but as the day progressed—and secondary attacks were attempted elsewhere—it became obvious that the potential for biological and chemical warfare conducted in American cities was a major concern for the military.

A little over three weeks after the World Trade Center attack, Florida state officials announced that they were treating a man for inhalation anthrax, the first such case reported in the United States in many years. Within days, there was a full-scale panic as other cases in New Jersey and New York surfaced. One report involved an assistant to NBC News anchor Tom Brokaw. The woman was exposed to the disease when she opened a letter from New Jersey that read:

> This is next
> Take Penacilin [*sic*] Now
> Death to America
> Death to Israel
> Allah is Great

When Florida officials announced that its anthrax patient, a photo editor at a tabloid newspaper, had died as a result of inhaled exposure to the disease, President Bush attempted to reassure the nation: "Thus far, it looks like a very isolated incident." Not feeling reassured was retired Fort Detrick researcher Bill Patrick, who knew a deliberate germ attack when he saw one. It was possible to get inhalation anthrax in nature, but the odds against it are so high as to be nonexistent. His immediate concern was that people exposed to the disease received prompt attention. "The earlier the treatment, the more people that you are going to save," he said during a NOVA interview. "For example, there is a very short window of treating [inhalation] anthrax. You've got to start treating exposed people within 24 to 48 hours of the exposure, before the overt symptoms of infection appear. Once the infection has generated a fever and you have shortness of breath, you can give all the antibiotics in the world, but the organism has released these toxins, and they kill you."[17]

There were more anthrax letters, resulting in more illnesses and deaths, but the overall threat evaporated as quickly as it had arisen. The more federal investigators looked into the matter, the more convinced they became that the instigator was someone who had intimate knowledge of anthrax—and not necessarily an Islamic terrorist.

Investigators soon focused their efforts on former employees from Fort Detrick, with Bill Patrick's name topping the list. Rumors that Patrick may have instigated the attack became so widespread that a BBC reporter set up an interview with him to ask that very question. "My goodness, I did not," Patrick answered. "I did not. . . . I'm an American patriot. . . . I want someone to be caught. I want the perpetrator to be caught, but I would rather think that it came from our enemies outside of our own country as opposed to our own people perpetrating this crime against our own."[18]

That Patrick would be considered a suspect is indicative of the paranoia sweeping the country at that time—and equally indicative of the power of germ warfare to inflict psychological damage on a defenseless and unsuspecting population. The person (or persons) who mailed the anthrax letters has never been apprehended and probably never will be held accountable for the deaths and illnesses the letters caused.

If there is a lesson to be learned from the anthrax letters, it is that anyone with a basic knowledge of scientific principles can build a deadly biological arsenal. On the day of his interview with NOVA reporters, Patrick staged an impromptu demonstration using a hand-pumped aerosol that sprayed a white powder into the air. He explained that seven and a half grams of anthrax could infect everyone in a fourteen-story building. When the nervous reporters asked what he was spraying, he told them that it was a stimulant powder that he had had manufactured for classroom demonstrations. He assured them that it was harmless.

*   *   *

The United States learned a great deal about biological warfare from the secret research conducted at Fort Detrick and from the Japanese experiments that took place during World War II. It learned that it could not develop a biological weapon without it eventually falling in the hands of its enemies. It learned that biological weapons, during their application, are just as dangerous to the users as they are to the intended targets. And it learned that defenses to biological warfare waged in the homeland will always be insufficient to prevent mass casualties.

Once the hopelessness of protecting the public against a biological attack is understood, it becomes obvious that the most potent weapon against an attack is an understanding of a potential enemy's motivation. Where the Bush administration has fallen short in its "war" against terrorism is in understanding the Islamic mind—and, until that happens, there can be no defense against terrorists who are willing to use weapons of mass destruction against American civilians. The administration explained the selection of the World Trade Center for attack by attributing it to a desire to destroy America's symbols of wealth and prosperity. That analysis was only partially true. The World Trade Center was highly symbolic to the Islamic terrorists who attacked it, but the precipitating symbolism did not extend to wealth and prosperity—the symbolism of the attack was not in destroying property but in using aircraft to kill large numbers of civilians. The American military used air power to bomb civilians in Germany during World War II and during the Vietnam War. The Islamic mind sees that as a cowardly way to wage battle. That is why suicide bombers are held in such high regard. Their mind-set is to do to America what America has done to others, using the same weapons. Very few American pilots died during the bombing of Germany and Vietnam, when compared with civilian deaths. An important part of the symbolism of the World Trade Center attack was that the Islamic "warriors" chose to die with their victims instead of remaining above it all, thus making them superior to their American enemies, which is no small matter in the Islamic world.

With a little thought, the Bush administration could anticipate the terrorists' next move by exploring the symbolism of specific weapons and targets. To the Islamic mind, symbolism is *everything*—both in religion and in everyday life. They will try to use nuclear weapons against the United States because it is the only country that has ever used nuclear weapons. They will try to use biological weapons against the American homeland because they feel that the US military has used biological and chemical weapons all over the world. Because of the importance of the emotionally charged symbolism of the event, they are likely to choose diseases that are historically linked to America—smallpox, anthrax, and yellow fever.

Of the three diseases, yellow fever is the most tempting, primarily because it already has terrorized the United States with the most deadly urban epidemics in history. It is the one disease that reeks with symbolism. It is true that there has not been a yellow fever epidemic in the United States for a century, but that is not because the disease has been wiped out. On the contrary, it continues to thrive in Africa and South America.

The most likely way for terrorists to introduce a yellow fever epidemic in America is by cultivating the disease in Africa or South America. (Detailed information on how to do that has been available in libraries, and now Web sites, for decades.) At that point, they have two options for bringing the disease to the United States: first, to breed mosquitoes for infection, as Walter Reed did in Cuba, and, second, to cultivate the disease in chicken eggs, as Bill Patrick did at Fort Detrick. It is more difficult to bring live mosquitoes into the United States than it is to bring infected eggs, but the logical place to enter with mosquitoes is at undefended sections of the US-Mexico border.

Since the United States imports about 96 million eggs a year,[19] shipping a few hundred infected eggs into the country poses little or no risk of detection. Once they are here, the live viruses can be used to aerosol yellow fever or other hemorrhagic fever viruses such as Ebola, Rift Valley fever, or Lassa fever.

Yellow fever was stopped a century ago at America's border because the mosquito problem was controlled by screened windows and doors, air conditioning, and spraying programs that systematically killed the insects at the source of their breeding grounds. Those very effective control measures offer little protection from a terrorist attack using either live mosquitoes or the disease in an aerosol.

Aerosol attacks can take place at movie theaters, shopping malls, or indoor and outdoor sporting events. All terrorists would have to do at indoor venues is attach the aerosol beneath their clothing and walk among their unsuspecting victims. If the terrorist "mules" have been vaccinated for yellow fever, then they can release the virus without worrying about contracting the disease themselves.

Outdoor venues offer the potential for a one-two punch that would allow them to follow up an aerosol attack with the release of live mosquitoes, both infected and noninfected. That scenario would go something like this: During the summer months, terrorists would target baseball games at either the student or professional level—and, during late summer and early fall months (anytime before the first frost), they would target football games. First, they would send vaccinated men or women with hidden aerosol containers up and down the aisles of the stands, perhaps holding hot dogs or soft drinks to look inconspicuous. That action alone would allow them to seed the audience with the disease. If the terrorists also released millions of infected mosquitoes in the vicinity of the sporting event, they could be assured of infecting a significant number of people, since whatever spraying the venue had done would have been finished well in advance of the event so as not to poison spectators.

At that point, every infected person becomes a potential weapon for the spread of the disease by attracting uninfected mosquitoes that pick up the virus after biting them and then transferring it to other unsuspecting persons. Since sports fans tend to be repeat customers, terrorists know that they will return to the scene of the infection within a week or two, thus making them targets for mosquitoes released in the vicinity of the sporting event in a second-wave attack.

With very little effort, a dozen well-trained terrorists could expose millions of Americans to the disease, and then quietly—and safely—fade back into anonymity. Once the attack has taken place, a chain reaction would begin that would be impossible to stop. According to a report from the twenty-six-member Working Group on Civilian Biodefense, published in the May 8, 2002, issue of the *Journal of the American Medical Association*, the American healthcare system is not ready for an attack by terrorists using yellow fever viruses—or any other virus in the hemorrhagic fever category. Said the authors of the report, led by Luciana Borio and Thomas Inglesby of Johns Hopkins University: "The diagnostic and therapeutic armamentarium urgently needs to be augmented. There also is an urgent need to develop vaccines and drug therapy."

The sad truth is that America has no defenses in place against a yellow fever attack—and can do very little once it begins. As far as detection at the border is concerned, the terrorists have the luxury of putting their brightest scientists up against low-level customs and immigration officials who may or may not have high school educations and who may or may not be motivated to do their jobs.

In 2001 Bill Patrick told his NOVA interviewers that he had been able to travel freely through all the major airports in the United States with his bag of noninfectious simulates and disseminators without ever once being stopped. Says Patrick: "And this concerns me. I would feel a lot more comfortable if someone were to challenge me. It brings home the point very, very dramatically that people who man these x-ray machines at airports and big buildings don't have a clue what to look for in terms of a [biological warfare] agent and a very simple disseminating device." Patrick's experiences occurred just before and after the World Trade Center attack, but there is no reason to think, even with all the security upgrades put in place at the airports since the attack, that situation has dramatically changed.

The CDC's Dr. Hayes is not convinced that terrorists would use hemorrhagic fever viruses such as yellow fever in an attack. "Somebody could bring in a crate of infected mosquitoes and let them go," says Hayes.[20] "That would seem like a complicated thing to do, but maybe there would be people who want to do that, I don't know." Other authorities are not so certain. Dr. Thomas W. McGovern, the former army major who was assigned to the Medical Research Institute of Infectious Diseases at Fort

Detrick and now has a private dermatology practice in Fort Wayne, Indiana, wrote in 1999 that "Filoviruses [a subgroup of hemorrhagic fever viruses] could make excellent offensive biologic warfare agents because they are highly infectious and deadly, and they can be stabilized for aerosol dissemination."[21]

Some researchers, not versed in the importance of symbolism to the terrorist mind, wonder why they would use yellow fever when they have easier options such as fungal toxins, which are more stable and easier to manufacture and offer multiple delivery options—or anthrax, which has proved its effectiveness. But to overlook the symbolism associated with yellow fever is to misunderstand the psychology involved in the selection process, especially among Muslims who build their lives around symbolism.

Yellow fever is a preferred weapon among Muslims because it is so engrained in American history and, from a historical perspective, represents the ultimate terror agent. Then, there is the matter of effectiveness. When yellow fever was rampant in the United States throughout the 1800s, the death toll held between 40 to 50 percent because many Americans had built up an acquired immunity to the disease, either as the result of childhood exposure or as the result of immigration from countries where yellow fever was prevalent. That would not be the case for epidemics today, when the percentage of Americans with acquired immunity is nearly zero. That is what makes yellow fever the ultimate death machine for terrorists.

At this point, the question arises: Have I just read a blueprint for terror? The answer is yes, but it is a blueprint that is readily available to terrorists on the Internet and in any big-city library. The purpose of publishing a blueprint like this is not to give ideas to terrorists—they already have the ideas and the means and knowledge to put them into action—but rather to alert the American public about the impending threat. With that in mind, the author recommends that citizens pressure authorities at local, state, and federal levels to close the loopholes in existing policies by:

- identifying the symbolic targets that are attractive to terrorists
- stopping all egg imports
- barring all aerosol containers on international and domestic flights
- installing virus-sensitive testing equipment at airports
- screening for aerosol containers at summer and fall sporting events
- increasing security at the Mexican and Canadian borders (customs and immigration agents should be educated about the threat posed by mosquitoes)
- supplying physicians with the latest information on diagnosing yellow fever
- increasing supplies of yellow fever vaccine.

Prevention is essential, since America is vulnerable once an attack begins. There is no cure for yellow fever, and it cannot be treated with antibiotics like, for example, anthrax can. Physicians can treat only the symptoms and ease the patient's pain and discomfort. The yellow fever vaccine is effective in preventing the disease, but there are dangers associated with it (it is risky for anyone over sixty years of age), and supplies are so low that only a selected few would be able to receive it. Asked if the United States could contain an epidemic in a city such as Miami, the CDC's Dr. Ned Hayes said, "I think we probably could, but it would be a challenge. These things always create a lot of public attention and concern. We would have to be right on top of it . . . but because of the [reasonably high] standard of living, I think we would have a reasonable chance of making sure it was a fairly small outbreak instead of an urban outbreak."

OTHER DISEASES YOU SHOULD KNOW ABOUT THAT CAN BE USED AS BIOLOGICAL WEAPONS

Trichothecene Mycotoxins

Trichothecene mycotoxins are a group of toxins that are produced by a common grain mold. They make excellent biological weapons because they are stable to work with and easy to produce in large quantities and can be dispersed in a number of different ways. They can be inhaled, ingested, or absorbed through the skin. They can invade the human body naturally through food contaminated with moldy grain.

Symptoms appear within sixty minutes, depending on the route of exposure. If inhaled, early symptoms will include sneezing, bloody and runny nose, wheezing, coughing, and bloody saliva. If eaten, early symptoms will include nausea and vomiting, stomach cramps, loss of appetite, and bloody diarrhea. If exposure is through the skin, early symptoms include burning or reddened skin, blistering, and the peeling away of large areas of skin. If contact was through the eyes, there will be blurred vision, pain, and redness. As the symptoms progress, blood pressure will drop, and there will be dizziness and fatigue, accompanied by an irregular heartbeat, and extensive bleeding.

Diagnosis is usually made on the basis of the symptoms and the results of blood and urine tests, although blood tests that identify trichothecene-specific antibodies have not been analytically validated. The most effective way to make a diagnosis is through the analysis of air samples, especially if patients report seeing smoke or "yellow rain." Unfortunately, there is no treatment for this infection. All physicians can do is treat the symptoms and hope for the best.

Smallpox

Smallpox is a serious infectious disease that is highly contagious from person to person. Once found throughout the world, it primarily struck children and young adults. Thanks to an effective nationwide vaccination campaign, smallpox became so rare in the United States by 1971 that physicians stopped giving vaccinations for it. By 1977, as the result of a massive vaccination program sponsored by the World Health Organization, the disease was effectively eradicated throughout the world, with the only remaining viruses existing in government research facilities. At one time, there was talk of destroying all samples of the virus, but that action was never taken for fear that terrorists might maintain their own samples.

Early symptoms include fever, malaise, headaches and body aches, and sometimes vomiting. The fever is usually in the 101-to-104 degree range. Two to four days after the early symptoms appear, a red rash emerges on the tongue and in the mouth. Those spots develop into sores that break open and spread large amounts of the virus into the mouth and throat. It is during this period that the person is the most contagious.

Around the time the sores in the mouth break down, a rash appears on the face and spreads to the arms and legs and then to the hands and feet. Typically, the rash spreads within twenty-four hours to all parts of the body. By the third day of the rash, raised bumps appear that are filled with a thick, opaque fluid that often has a depression in the center that looks like a human naval. Soon the bumps transform into pustules that form a crust and then a scab. By the end of the second week after the rash appears, most of the sores have scabbed over. After about six days, the scabs fall off, leaving marks on the skin that transform into pitted scars. Once the scabs have fallen off, the person is no longer contagious.

If smallpox is diagnosed within one to four days of exposure, the smallpox vaccination is sometimes effective in preventing the illness or lessening the severity of the illness. Once the disease takes hold, treatment is limited, since there is no smallpox-specific medication. Patients are isolated and made comfortable, and sometimes antibiotics are given to combat secondary infections.

There are two forms of smallpox—Variola major, which has a mortality rate of about 30 percent, and Variola minor, which has a mortality rate of less than 1 percent. If used by terrorists, the virus would probably be released in aerosol form, which would enable it to remain viable for as long as twenty-four hours.

Anthrax

Anthrax is a bacterium whose spores can cause serious illness. Until anthrax spores were sent through the mail in 2001 by persons unknown, there had not been a case of inhalational anthrax in the United States for more than twenty years. What little physicians know about inhalation anthrax is the result of an outbreak in 1979 at a military facility in Russia. Seventy-nine cases were reported, with sixty-eight deaths.

There are three ways to contract anthrax—through the skin, through contaminated food, and through airborne spores that enter the lungs. It cannot be passed from person to person. Death rates are 90 to 100 percent for anthrax that has been inhaled, but lower for anthrax that enters the body through food and the skin. Anthrax spores are tasteless and invisible to the naked eye, but thousands of them can reside on the head of a pin.

Initial symptoms of inhalational anthrax resemble those of the common cold—sore throat, mild fever, muscle aches, and malaise. However, after several days, the disease can progress to severe breathing problems and shock. Initial symptoms of gastrointestinal anthrax include nausea, loss of appetite, and vomiting, followed by abdominal pain, severe diarrhea, and the vomiting of blood. This type of antrax results in death in 25 to 60 percent of cases. Initial symptoms of cutaneous anthrax (through the skin) include raised, itchy bumps that resemble insect bites. Within a day or so, a painless ulcer with a black area in the center will appear. Death occurs in only about 20 percent of these cases.

Treatment can be successful if the disease is quickly diagnosed, but that could be a problem in the event of a biological attack, since few American physicians have any clinical experience with the disease. Antibiotics are recommended, but their success depends on how quickly they are administered after the infection has taken place. Recommended antibiotics include penicillin, doxycycline (for penicillin-sensitive patients), and erythromycins. A new drug, ciprofloxacin (Cipro), was recommended by the Food and Drug Administration in the wake of the 2001 attack, but since then the drug has come under criticism because of reports of serious side effects, including complete liver and kidney failure.

Botulism

Mention botulism and most people think of mother's advice not to eat food, especially green beans, that comes from cans that show signs of damage or swelling. But there is more to the disease than that. Botulism is caused by a potent toxin that can severely damage nerves and cause paralysis that ends in death. It is found in nature in the form of spores that can exist in a dormant state for many years. It is not until moisture and nutrients are present—and oxygen is absent (the reason canned food is a frequent incubator)—that the spores can grow and produce deadly toxins. The most common causes of botulism are associated with canned food, but it is possible to get the disease by inhaling small amounts of dust or from a contaminated wound.

Symptoms of food-borne botulism typically develop suddenly, within eighteen to thirty-six hours of exposure. The more toxins that are eaten, the faster the symptoms will appear. There have been cases in which people have displayed symptoms within four hours of eating the contaminated food. In adults, early symptoms include constipation, nausea, and vomiting. (For infants, the main symptoms are poor feeding and lethargy.) As the disease progresses, the victim experiences weakness or paralysis, beginning with the head muscles and progressing down the body. Breathing becomes difficult. Without treatment, death is very likely. The symptoms for botulism acquired through a wound are similar to the symptoms for food-borne exposure, except the gastrointestinal symptoms often will be absent.

Treatment consists of antitoxins to block the progression of the disease, induced vomiting to rid the body of any remaining toxins in the stomach, and laxatives. Beyond those treatments, there is not much physicians can do, except make the patient comfortable. Antibiotics are not used, since they are ineffective. The biggest problem that a victim may face early on is simply finding a physician who can diagnosis the disease. It is frequently misdiagnosed as stroke or a variety of other diseases that cause muscle weakness. Diagnosis is enhanced if more than one person from the same family or group comes in for treatment. The diagnosis can be confirmed by testing for toxins in the blood. If the victim is lucky enough to recover from this disease, he or she may face many years of tiredness and shortness of breath.

Tularemia

Tularemia is caused by bacteria usually associated with rural areas. It has been reported in every state in the United States, except Hawaii, but it is most common in Arkansas, Missouri, Oklahoma, Kansas, South Dakota, Montana, and on Martha's Vineyard. It is carried by a variety of small animals, including rats, squirrels, rabbits, and muskrats. It is sometimes called rabbit fever.

This disease passes from animal to human by way of insects such as mosquitoes, ticks, and flies, but humans also can get the disease by eating meat from infected animals, from infected water, or from dust that has been created by sweeping areas where infected animals have lived. Tularemia cannot be passed from person to person. The United States made weapons in the 1950s and 1960s that could spray the disease, but they were supposedly all destroyed by the early 1970s. Other countries—and terrorists—may have stockpiles of the disease for use as offensive weapons.

There are six types of tularemia and the symptoms depend on the type:

- Ulceroglandular, the most common type, is caused by the bite of a tick. Early symptoms include a sore that does not heal (the site of the tick bite). The sore will develop into an ulcer that has a black base. Adults typically experience swollen glands, accompanied by chills, headache, and fever.
- Glandular, the second most common type, presents symptoms of fever and swollen glands, but no evidence of an ulcer.
- Typhoidal, caused by inhalation of the bacteria, displays symptoms that begin with extreme tiredness and fever and escalates into pneumonia. Glands are not swollen with this type.
- Oculoglandular, which is caused by the bacteria entering the body through the eyes, typically gets it start when the victim touches his or her eyes after coming into contact with the bacteria. The first symptom may be an infection that is confined to one eye. Pus will ooze from the eye, and neck glands will be swollen.
- Oropharyngeal, which enters through the mouth or throat, will first show symptoms as a sore throat that produces a large amount of phlegm.
- Pneumonic, which can be caused by inhaling the bacteria, sometimes accompanies another type of tularemia. It symptoms are similar to those produced by oropharyngeal and typhoidal tularemia.

Treatment usually consists of antibiotics such as streptomycin and treatment of specific symptoms such as fever and breathing difficulties. There is a vaccine for tularemia, but it is not widely available, and it is of no use once exposure to the bacteria has occurred. In the event of a biological attack, symptoms would appear between one to fourteen days after exposure. About one-third of untreated people die, but death rarely occurs among people who have received proper treatment.

Ebola

Ebola is a virus from the hemorrhagic fever family that has occurred mostly in Africa, which is why the various strains of the virus have African names such as Ebola Zaire or Ebola Sudan. In nature, the disease is spread through contact with infected animals or by contact with the blood of an infected person. The incubation of the disease ranges from two to twenty-one days.

Symptoms begin with chills, muscle aches, loss of appetite, diarrhea, sore throat, and headaches. As the disease progresses, there will be bleeding from the nose, vomiting, rash, and broken blood vessels in the eyes, followed by chest pain, shock, and death. Psychologically, it is a frightening disease because as it progresses, medical personnel wear more and more protective gear, beginning with masks and gloves and quickly proceeding to gowns and goggles. It is a disease that precludes human contact.

There is no specific treatment for Ebola. It consists of supportive therapy such as intravenous fluids, oxygen, and blood-pressure control. Ebola Zaire is fatal in about 90 percent of the cases, but Ebola Sudan is fatal in only about 60 percent of the cases. Death usually occurs within ten days of the appearance of symptoms.

If terrorists launched an attack with Ebola, the US healthcare system would be poorly prepared to respond, according to the twenty-six-member Working Group on Civilian Biodefense, which identified an "urgent need to develop vaccines and drug therapy."[22]

Bubonic Plague

Bubonic plague is one of those diseases that you read about in history books but never give thought to in real life. It is transmitted to humans by flea bites from rodents or by the ingestion of feces of infected fleas. It also can be spread in the air by victims who cough infected droplets that are inhaled by healthy people.

Symptoms include the sudden onset of a high fever, muscular pains, severe headaches, chills, seizures, and swollen lymph glands in the groin, armpits, or neck. The most common area of swelling is in the groin.

Treatment consists of antibiotics such as streptomycin or tetracycline, oxygen, and intravenous fluids. Victims are isolated from other patients, and their family and friends are given antibiotics as a preventive measure. Half of all victims die if not treated.

CHAPTER SEVEN

global warming casts ominous shadow

The earth's atmosphere performs like the walls and roof of a greenhouse, allowing sunlight to enter, but preventing heat from escaping. As sunlight passes through the "roof" and heats the earth's surface, it gives off infrared radiation that travels back toward the atmosphere. Instead of escaping into space, some of the radiation is trapped by "greenhouse" gases such as ozone and carbon dioxide, which send the radiation back to the earth's surface, creating a wide range of effects, including extreme weather, a rise in temperature, and rising sea levels. That process is called global warming.

For most of the earth's existence, global warming has not been an issue. The most notable exception, of course, may be the extinction of dinosaurs at the end of the Cretaceous geologic period, about 60 million years ago. No one knows for certain why that happened. One theory is that the elevation of the Rocky Mountain chain, which occurred during that time period, resulted in the drainage of the swamps and lowlands on which the dinosaurs were dependent for food. Another theory has it that a huge asteroid hit the earth and created a monstrous black cloud that hung in the atmosphere long enough to create a magnified global warming effect, thus wiping out most of the life on the planet. Whatever the reasons for global warming in the past, it

225

has little to do with global warming of the future, for, barring another devastating asteroid strike, humans—and humans alone—will bear that responsibility.

It took all of human history for earth's population to reach a billion and a half people by 1900, but in the one hundred years since then, the earth's population has added that many new people every thirty-three years so that today we looking at a population of 6.5 billion, with the vast majority of this growth happening in the developing world.

Population is an important ingredient in global warming, not just because humans produce carbon dioxide with each breath of life, but because the enormous support systems that humans have created to make life safer and more enjoyable are the major contributors to global warming. That is because worldwide economic development has resulted in increased carbon dioxide production with the burning of fossil fuels, which releases carbon dioxide into the atmosphere, and the massive clearing of forests, which reduces nature's ability to convert carbon dioxide into people-friendly oxygen. Today, the major producers of carbon dioxide are power plants (33 percent), factories and home heating (33 percent), automobiles (22 percent), and airplanes and railway (12 percent).[1]

Twenty-five years ago, scientists began sounding an alarm about the potentially catastrophic results of global warming, but governments have been slow to respond, especially the United States, where corporations involved in enterprises that produce carbon dioxide and other pollutants exert considerable control over the political process.

Thus far, the primary proponent of reversing global warming has been the Intergovernmental Panel of Climate Change (IPCC), an organization composed of thousands of scientists from around the world who provide updates on the progression of global warming. The IPCC has come under attack from right-wing, political-action groups that do not believe that global warming exists and see a left-wing conspiracy in efforts to diminish pollutants in the atmosphere, but the organization has been endorsed by the US National Academy of Sciences, which saw no evidence of political bias in the organization's investigative process and assessments.[2]

The evidence put forward by the IPCC and other organizations is chilling:

- Warming in the twentieth century is greater today than at any time in the past four hundred years.
- The earth's mean surface temperature has increased by about 1.1° Fahrenheit.
- Seven of the warmest years in the twentieth century occurred in the 1990s. So far, 2001 was the second hottest year overall, even though its winter took first place.
- Arctic ice has lost about 40 percent of its thickness over the past forty years.
- A growing number of studies show plants and animals changing their range and behavior in response to shifts in climate.

"In part because of fossil fuel use in the twentieth century, carbon dioxide in the atmosphere is now at its highest level in 420,000 years," wrote James Gustave Speth in *America and the Crisis of the Global Environment.* "While the public in the United States and especially abroad is increasingly aware of this issue, few Americans appreciate how close at hand is the widespread loss of the American landscape. The best current estimate is that, unless there is a major world correction, climate change projected for late this century will make it impossible for about half the American land to sustain the types of plants and animals now on that land. A huge portion of American's protected areas—everything from wooded lands held by community conservancies to our national parks, forests and wilderness—is threatened. In one projection, the much-loved maple-beech-birch forests of New England simply disappear off the U.S. map. In another, the Southeast becomes a huge grassland and savanna unable to support forests because it is too hot and dry."

In many respects, America has the most to lose because of global warming, yet US political leadership has consistently blocked efforts to do anything about the problem, a result of corporate opposition to actions that could affect profits. The 1997 Kyoto Protocol to the Convention on Climate Change was the first international treaty to propose specific remedies. Basically, it requires that industrial nations reduce, by 2010, their greenhouse gas emissions to a level below that of 1990.

To the bafflement of other industrial nations, the Bush administration rejected the Kyoto Protocol, a decision that prompted both domestic and international criticism. Instead, the administration referred the matter to the National Academy of Sciences, which, to the administration's surprise, found agreement with the protocol's key provisions. In brief, the NAS report, titled *Climate Change Science: An Analysis of Some Key Questions,* concluded that:

- Greenhouse gases are accumulating in earth's atmosphere as a result of human activities, causing temperatures to rise. Global average temperatures warmed by about 1° F in the twentieth century and could increase by 2.5° to 10.5° F in this century.
- Human-induced warming and sea-level rising are expected to continue throughout this century and into the next.
- This warming is caused by the cumulative effects of several greenhouse gases that have built up steadily in the atmosphere, including carbon dioxide from fossil fuel combustion and deforestation, methane from fossil fuels and agricultural activities, nitrous oxide from agricultural activities and the chemical industry, and specialty chemicals including CFCs.

- Global warming could well have serious adverse societal and ecological impacts by the end of this century, and temperature and sea levels could also continue to rise well into the next century even if societies stabilize the levels of greenhouse gases in the atmosphere.[3]

The White House letter that initiated the NAS report was brief: "The Administration is conducting a review of U.S. policy on climate change. We seek the Academy's assistance in identifying the areas in the science of climate change where there are the greatest certainties and uncertainties. We would also like your views on whether there are any substantive differences between the IPCC Reports and the IPCC summaries."

The NAS response to the latter request came as a surprise to the White House:

The committee finds that the full IPCC Working Group I report is an admirable summary of research activities in climate science, and the full report is adequately summarized in the *Technical Summary*. The full WGI report and its *Technical Summary* are not specifically directed at policy. . . . It is critical that the IPCC process remain truly representative of the scientific community. The committee's concerns focus primarily on whether the process is likely to become less representative in the future because of the growing voluntary time commitment required to participate as a lead or coordinating author and the potential that the scientific process will be viewed as being too heavily influenced by governments which have specific postures with regard to treaties, emission controls and other policy instruments. The United States should promote actions that improve the IPCC process while also ensuring that its strengths are maintained.[4]

Four years later, in July 2005, when President George W. Bush attended a summit of big industrial nations in Scotland, commonly referred to as the Group of 8, he refused to support the group's efforts to address global warming. "I recognize that the surface of the earth is warmer and that an increase in greenhouse gases caused by humans is contributing to the problem," he said at a press conference. But he added that he wanted to depart from the thinking behind the Kyoto Protocol, which already had been ratified by the other Group of 8 nations: "The reason it didn't work for the world is many developing nations weren't included in Kyoto. I've also told our friends in Europe that Kyoto would have wrecked our economy. I don't see how you can be president of the United States and agree to an agreement that would have put a lot of people out of work."[5]

*   *   *

One aspect of global warming that has received little notice is the effect that even a minor temperature change will have on the worldwide spread of infectious diseases, but particularly in North America. The history of yellow fever epidemics is that they have appeared throughout the South and Southeast, but only in port cities in the North, where their entry was linked to ships arriving from the Caribbean or Africa. A continuation of the rising temperatures that we are experiencing today will have a profound effect on northern states and Canada, as increased summer heat draws mosquitoes northward to areas that have little experience combating the insect.

In 1999, the World Health Organization (WHO) issued a warning that North America was not the only area at risk. Also at risk, says WHO, are Britain and the rest of Europe, where the average temperature has increased by nearly 1° centigrade. The rate of increase is so steep, WHO concluded, that the average global temperature would rise by another 3.5° by the year 2100. Accompanying that increase would be changes in rainfall, which would result in new areas of flooding and increased humidity, an insect's best friend because these conditions offer a more hospitable environment in which to breed.

Paul R. Epstein, associate director of the Center for Health and the Global Environment at Harvard Medical School, wrote an article for *Scientific American* in 2000 in which he concluded that global warming could have a profound effect on humans. "That prospect is deeply troubling, because infectious illness is a genie that can be very hard to put back into its bottle," he wrote. "It may kill fewer people in one fell swoop than a raging flood or an extended drought, but once it takes root in a community, it often defies eradication and can invade other areas."

A 2002 study conducted by researchers at Princeton University and Cornell University concluded that climate warming is allowing disease-carrying viruses such as yellow fever to invade North America. As a result, the researchers warn that yellow fever and other related diseases could become more common as milder winters allow the seasonal survival of more mosquitoes. A warmer climate also could enable mosquitoes to move into areas once protected by cold weather. "In all the discussion about climate change, this has really been kind of left out," said Drew Harvell, a Cornell University marine ecologist and lead author of the study. "Just a one-or-two-degree change in temperature can lead to disease outbreaks."

The comprehensive two-year study, developed by the National Center for Ecological Analysis and Synthesis, is the first to look at disease in terms of global warming. Said Harvell: "What is most surprising is the fact that climate sensitive outbreaks are happening with so many different types of pathogens—viruses, bacteria, fungi and parasites—as well as in such a wide range of hosts including corals, oysters, terrestrial plants, birds and humans." Added coauthor Richard Ostfeld, from the Institute of Ecosystem Studies in Millbrook, New York: "This isn't just a question of coral bleaching for a few marine ecologists, nor just a question of malaria for a few health officials—the number of similar increases in disease incidence is astonishing. We don't want to be alarmist, but we are alarmed."[6] Andrew Dobson, a Princeton epidemiologist associated with the study, says the risk for humans is going up: "The diseases we should be most worried about are the vector [insect] transmitted diseases." Even with small temperature increases, he concludes, natural ecosystems are disrupted in such a way as to create more fertile habitats for infectious diseases such a malaria and yellow fever.

Among those individuals not convinced that global warming will bring diseases such as yellow fever into the United States is the CDC's Ned Hayes, which, according to one's point of view, is either comforting or highly disturbing. Hayes thinks that a yellow fever epidemic caused by global warming, as opposed to one caused by terrorists, has little chance of getting a foothold in the United States because of the country's high socioeconomic level and because of the prevalence of window screens and air conditioning. Says Hayes:

> The possibility of getting a major urban yellow fever epidemic in the continental U.S. is relatively low. San Juan, Puerto Rico is different. There is more potential for problems there than on the mainland U.S. In 2000, we studied a dengue [outbreak] on the Mexican-U.S. border. Dengue, as you may know is transmitted by the same vector [mosquito family]. There was an outbreak of dengue in Mexico and a few cases in Laredo on the U.S. side. The two areas were almost identical. The only division between the two places is the Rio Grande and yet you have a high prevalence on the Mexican side and virtually no transmission on the U.S. side. When we looked at the populations of mosquitoes there were plenty of mosquitoes on the Texas side, high enough density to support epidemic transmission. So why did that not occur? We did a survey and it was what you would expect—the difference in the socio-economic conditions. It's not the climate that's influencing whether we have dengue or yellow fever—it's the living conditions.[7]

Not in agreement with Hayes are the researchers who conducted a 1998 study funded by the Climate Policy and Assessment

Division of the EPA, the National Institute of Public Health, and the Center for Medical, Agricultural, and Veterinary Entomology of the US Department of Agriculture. Using computers to simulate the circulation of the earth's climate, the researchers predicted that rising temperatures will increase the range of a mosquito that transmits the dengue fever virus. All three computer models used by the researchers indicated that dengue's epidemic potential increases with a relatively small temperature rise. At risk are the United States and all other countries around the world that are located in temperate zones, especially those that border on endemic areas where the disease is currently prevalent. "Since inhabitants of these border regions would lack immunity from past exposures, dengue fever transmission among these new populations could be extensive," says Jonathan Patz, lead author for the report and a physician at Johns Hopkins School of Public Health.[8] "Our study makes no claim that climate factors are the most important determinants of dengue fever. However, our computer models illustrate that climate change may have a substantial global impact on the spread of dengue fever."

Perhaps the best method of determining the effect of global warming on yellow fever is to examine the effect that warmer temperatures are having on related mosquito-borne diseases such as dengue, malaria, West Nile fever, and encephalitis. If they show signs of increased incidence, then it is only a matter of time before the yellow fever virus makes its reappearance.

Paul R. Epstein, associate director of the Center for Health and the Global Environment at Harvard, feels that those diseases are going to become more prevalent because of the mosquito's sensitivity to meteorological conditions. "Cold can be a friend to humans," he writes, "because it limits mosquitoes to seasons and regions where temperatures stay above certain minimums. Winter freezing kills many eggs, larvae and adults outright . . . within their survivable range of temperatures, mosquitoes proliferate faster and bite more as the air becomes warmer. At the same time, greater heat speeds the rate at which pathogens inside them reproduce and mature. . . . As whole areas heat up, then, mosquitoes could expand into formerly forbidden territories, bringing illness with them."[9]

One of the most disturbing developments in recent years has been the arrival of the West Nile virus. In August 1999, tissue samples from a dead crow found in the New York City area and from a horse that died of a central nervous system disease on Long Island, New York, were sent to the National Veterinary Services Laboratories in Ames, Iowa, for identification. Meanwhile, more than two dozen cases of suspicious equine illness were identified in Suffolk and Nassau Counties on Long Island.

By September, the Centers for Disease Control and Prevention was able to identify the infected tissue samples as hosts to West Nile virus, a disease first isolated in 1937 in Africa and the Middle East. It is closely related to St. Louis encephalitis, which is indigenous to the United States and Canada, but, as of August 1999, West Nile virus had never been isolated in tissue samples in North America.

Accompanying the deaths of dozens of horses and thousands of birds in the New York City area was an outbreak of human encephalitis that baffled health officials because it appeared to be a new strain. As the human death toll rose, genetic sequencing studies revealed that humans, birds, and horses were all infected by the same strain of West Nile, one that showed strong similarities to isolates from the Middle East.

Almost right away, the disease, which is spread from animals to humans by mosquitoes, began moving from New York to New Jersey and Connecticut, where eighty-three cases of West Nile were reported within one year. By 2005 the disease had spread all the way to California, infecting humans in almost every state except Maine, Alaska, and Hawaii. At greatest risk are those people over fifty years of age.

"Yellow fever is transmitted from human to mosquito to

human, but with West Nile the reservoir of infection is the birds and possibly some reptiles and you have a different dynamic—humans are sort of incidental," says Dr. Ned Hayes. "You don't get human to human transmission with West Nile. The disease has spread east to west, north to south, going to both Canada and Mexico, but we still don't know what's going to happen in the United States. It is possible it could continue to cause locally intense epidemics in certain parts of the country, and it's also possible it might take a course like St. Louis encephalitis, which flares up after years of dormancy."[10]

Most of the humans infected with West Nile have no symptoms, and the death rate is only one out of one thousand infections, but it can be a devastating disease to those who develop paralysis. Early symptoms include fever, headache, nausea, vomiting, rashes, muscle weakness, and swollen lymph nodes. There is no treatment specific to West Nile, and there is no vaccine available to provide protection. Physicians have limited options for the treatment of severe cases—hospitalization, the use of intravenous fluids and nutrition, respiratory support, good nursing care, and the use of antibiotics to prevent secondary infections. Those who recover from the illness do so because of their immune systems and not because of medical treatment.

West Nile is of interest to yellow fever researchers because it demonstrates the speed with which a mosquito-induced disease can spread from state to state within a relatively brief period. Since West Nile can be spread only from animal to human, it is a friendlier disease, epidemically speaking, than yellow fever, which can spread with lightning speed from mosquito to human to mosquito to human. For those concerned about the reemergence of yellow fever in the United States, West Nile's unhindered march across the heartland offers little in the way of comfort.[11]

Malaria is another mosquito-related disease that is raising red flags. Each year the disease kills more than three thousand people, mostly children. Some scientists predict that, by the end of this century, the zone of malaria transmission will increase from one containing 45 percent of the world's population to one containing 60 percent. Malaria has a long history in the United States, but public health measures throughout the country were successful in isolating the disease and restricting it to California by the 1980s. As temperatures have risen since then, the threat has increased the incidence of malaria. In recent years, outbreaks have occurred in Florida, Texas, Georgia, Michigan, New Jersey, New York, and, to the surprise of many, Toronto, Canada.

Similarly, St. Louis encephalitis, a flavivirus related to Japanese encephalitis, has shown gains in recent years, with record spikes in the 1990s, which, incidentally, were the hottest years of this century. In the summer of 1999, New York City experienced an outbreak of encephalitis that killed a number of people. Normally, encephalitis, which causes inflammation of the brain, can effectively be treated, but the survival odds are lessened for those with weakened immune systems or for senior citizens.

At the time of the New York outbreak, Dr. Cathey Falvo, director for International and Public Health at New York Medical College, was concerned whether the increased temperatures would allow the disease to survive the winter. Falvo was particularly concerned about the effect that global warming was having on increased incidence of the disease. If global warming continues on its present course, she said, milder winters will result that will not be cold enough to kill the microbes, thus allowing the organisms to still be around when mosquitoes again become active in the spring.[12]

The same year that the disease appeared in New York, it also showed up in New Orleans, with twenty reported cases. Four years later, in 2003, St. Louis encephalitis was reported in Washington State, which had not had a case in over thirty years. The man who was diagnosed with the disease recovered, but it alarmed health officials who already were preparing for a West Nile virus outbreak.

CHAPTER EIGHT

the disease that won't go away

In spring 2002, before leaving for Brazil on a fishing trip to the Rio Negro River in the Amazon River Basin, Tom McCullough, a forty-seven-year-old oil and gas executive with LMP Petroleum of Corpus Christi, Texas, somehow overlooked the advice on the outfitter's Web site that stated: "The international medical community suggests yellow fever and malaria prophylaxis for the Amazon region. This is not a requirement to enter Brazil, but merely a suggestion."

McCullough may have not taken that advice seriously because the travel agent's brochure put the yellow fever danger in less threatening terms: "We do not suggest any inoculations of any kind for this trip . . . but to make sure you are worry free, consult with your personal physician."

Of the fifteen Texans who made the trip, eight were appropriately vaccinated for yellow fever, according to World Health Organization guidelines—and of the seven who were not vaccinated, one man had received the vaccine eleven years earlier (one year beyond WHO recommendations), and one had been vaccinated less than a week before arrival in Brazil (ten days is recommended).

For the five men who rolled the dice, the payoff must have seemed worth the risk: The Rio Negro River is a spectacular waterway that travels parallel to the Amazon River for more than twenty kilometers before the two waterways merge, offering spectacular fishing opportunities for countless species of trophy fish, including the much-sought-after peacock bass.

Most of the boats, or "gaiolas" as they are called by natives, on the Rio Negro are small, crudely constructed vessels that typically have hammocks strung across the decks, but the Corpus Christi executives traveled in style aboard an air-conditioned yacht, which allowed them to sleep comfortably in plush accommodations that afforded nighttime protection from mosquitoes. Once they reached a prime fishing site, the travelers broke up into smaller groups and fished the river in motorized bass boats of the type seen in lakes and rivers all across America. For protection against mosquitoes, the men all wore clothing that had been impregnated with DEET.

By all accounts, it was a successful fishing trip. The men returned to Texas with enough fish stories to amaze even the most dedicated non-Amazon fisherman. However, within days of his arrival back in Texas, McCullough complained that he did not feel well. After four days of abdominal pain and headaches, including a one-day bout of fever of 102.8°, he went to the emergency room of a local hospital, where he was treated for his symptoms and discharged.

Once he returned home, his high fever continued, and his condition worsened.

"What is happening to me?" he repeatedly asked his wife, Stephanie.

Two days later, Stephanie took him back to the hospital with a new symptom—intractable vomiting. Bacterial cultures of his blood, urine, and spinal fluid were negative, and a malaria smear was, too. Not until the results of the liver function test came back did doctors understand the seriousness of his condition. Two test results were especially alarming: His alanine transaminase (ALT) reading was 7,600 (normal is 30–65), and his aspartate transaminase (AST) was 13,700 (normal is 15–37). (These tests measure enzyme function and can indicate a serious problem.) McCullough was asked by doctors if he recalled being bitten by a mosquito; he said that he did not remember that happening.

Within three days after admission to the hospital, McCullough developed shock and seizures. Sitting at his bedside, Stephanie prayed that her husband wouldn't die before St. Patrick's Day, his favorite holiday. He died on the fourth day, just an hour and a half before March 17, leaving behind a wife who was stunned by the suddenness and senselessness of her husband's death.

Local doctors were baffled by the progression of the disease. Everything that could go wrong with a human body took place with alarming speed, generating one organ failure after another. Once the death was reported to the Centers for Disease Control and Prevention, the agency ran tests on the serum samples collected during McCullough's stay in the hospital. Tests using samples taken the second day of the illness were negative for St. Louis encephalitis, Venezuelan equine viruses, dengue, and yellow fever. However, tests run on blood samples collected three to seven days after symptoms appeared, and on a postmortem liver sample, revealed the presence of the yellow fever virus.

McCullough died without ever knowing the cause of his illness. At it turned out, he was the only person in his fishing group to contract yellow fever. Later, questioned by reporters about her husband's death, Stephanie said that he was never been advised of the possibility of a yellow fever threat before leaving for Brazil. The other members of his group who had not been vaccinated, when interviewed by health department investigators, admitted that they had been "unconcerned" about a yellow fever danger.

Why was Tom McCullough the only person on that fishing trip to die? Once precautions were tossed to the wind, it became a matter of luck. It was left to an infectious disease technician with the Texas health department to put it in perspective: "One mosquito bite can kill you. There's a bazillion mosquitoes and if only one has yellow fever, there you go."[1]

Tom McCullough was not the only unlucky man in America, not by any means. Three years earlier, a previously healthy forty-eight-year-old man showed up at the emergency room of a California hospital, complaining of fever, joint pain, nausea, abdominal pain, and vomiting. He told doctors that he has just returned for a ten-day trip with six friends to the rainforests of Venezuela.

Suspicious that his patient could be suffering from a viral hemorrhagic fever, the emergency room doctor contacted state health department officials. Within three days, the patient experienced seizures and developed upper respiratory obstruction, after which he was placed on mechanical ventilation and transferred to the intensive care unit. Blood and urine cultures were negative for malaria and bacteria pathology. His condition, complicated by cardiac arrhythmias, deteriorated rapidly, and he died within days.

An autopsy of the chest and abdomen, performed at the University of California San Francisco Medical Center, showed yellow fever viral antigens in the patient's liver. Liver enzyme tests disclosed that he had AST and ALT scores in the 5,000 range, a clear indication of organ failure. A follow-up investigation by health department officials revealed that the patient had received vaccinations before leaving for Venezuela for hepatitis A, malaria, tetanus, and typhoid, but not yellow fever. However, five of his traveling companions did receive yellow fever vaccinations. Like Tom McCullough, the patient used DEET-based mosquito repellents, but unlike McCullough, he reported numerous mosquito bites while on the trip.[2]

Three years previously, a Tennessee man returned from a nine-day trip to Brazil complaining of fever and headache. He died within ten days of the onset of symptoms, and the yellow fever virus was identified by an examination of tissue samples. These are isolated cases, to be sure, but they are indicative of a growing threat to America, signal flares that are ignored at everyone's peril.

*   *   *

In South America, yellow fever currently is rampant in all of Colombia (except its western edge); all of Venezuela, Trinidad and Tobago, Guyana, Suriname, French Guiana, Ecuador; and Peru (except for the coastal areas); eastern Bolivia; the northern tip of Argentina, where it adjoins Brazil and Paraguay; and Panama. In Africa, yellow fever is present in thirty-three countries, which have a combined population of 508 million; most at risk of infection are those who live or travel within a band from 15° north to 10° south of the equator. Travelers going to the following locations should take special precautions: the northern border of Senegal, extreme southern Mauritania, southern Mali, southern Niger, central Chad, southern Sudan, the northern border of Ethiopia, and southern Somalia and the central coastal region. If you have traveled to a country that is infected with yellow fever, most other countries will require you to show an International Certificate of Vaccination as proof that you were vaccinated prior to your trip to an infected country. Without a certificate, you may be denied entry to some countries, including your homeland.

Brazil, which today accounts for 25 percent of all yellow fever cases reported from South America,[3] has always been a troublesome source of the disease. There has been an ongoing battle to eliminate the disease since 1923, when the Rockefeller Foundation accepted an invitation to tackle the yellow fever problem in that country and sent Dr. Joseph White, a veteran of the 1905 epidemic in New Orleans. White supervised antimosquito campaigns in all the major cities between Rio de Janeiro and Manaos, an inland port in the Amazon Valley—and, generally, witnessed good results. By 1925 the disease had dwindled to a level that led researchers of that era to believe that the end of yellow fever was in sight for the American continent.[4]

By 1937 it was obvious to everyone involved in public health issues that yellow fever was not going to go quietly into the night.

In a speech delivered at the American Public Health Association in New Orleans, Dr. Fred L. Soper, the then-current administrator of the Rockefeller Foundation effort in Brazil, said: "The extent to which present beliefs regarding the epidemiology of yellow fever differ from those of just a few years ago is not generally known outside of the small group of workers actively engaged in the study and control of this disease. It must come as a great surprise to the majority of the members of the American Public Health Association . . . to learn that the epidemiology of yellow fever is still a sufficiently important problem to merit a place on a program devoted to public health problems of immediate interest to health workers in the United States." Soper went on to say that from 1926, when the Rockefeller Foundation made a major effort to rid Brazil of the disease, to 1936, the year of his address, healthcare workers lived in an "age of disillusion and partial enlightenment."[5]

Soper's point was that yellow fever is a disease that simply will not go away. To his dismay, he pointed out that the control methods used with success in the United States were inadequate for South America. "Yellow fever does not invariably disappear when the *Aedes aegytpi* mosquito is sufficiently controlled, and the duration of infection in many districts is not dependent upon the introduction of non-immune human elements into these districts," he said. "Yellow fever may occur under a great variety of conditions, and the factors determining its occurrence are in large part still undetermined."[6]

Soper made the point to his public health colleagues that simply knocking down mosquitoes during a one- or two-year period was not enough to eradicate the disease. It can appear to be gone one year—indeed, for a number of years—and then reappear with a vengeance without warning. Soper's focus was Brazil and South America, but his conclusions, made all those years ago, are equally valid for the United States.

Dr. Ned Hayes, a medical epidemiologist with the viral disease branch of CDC, says that America maintains ties with health ministries in the infected countries so that the continuing yellow fever threat can be monitored. "We try to work with them to analyze those cases and determine increased areas of risk," he says. "There has been a long time since there were any reports of yellow fever in Central America, but there appear to be many cases reported in South America. We work with the Pan American health organizations to provide assistance to South America, if asked. Urban yellow fever has not been described in Central America in a long while, but if the threat were to happen, that would be an international health emergency. The surveillance data that we look at from Latin America helps us better determine where the areas of risk are for travelers from the United States."[7]

Each year, according to the World Health Organization, there are an estimated two hundred thousand cases of yellow fever worldwide that generate thirty thousand deaths: Given the likelihood that other cases have occurred but not been detected, one confirmed case of yellow fever is considered by medical authorities to be an outbreak. One of the problems faced by currently infected countries is that few have national laboratories where yellow fever blood tests can be performed—and that means that many cases slip through the surveillance system and result in incorrect diagnoses.

*   *   *

Yellow fever is an infectious viral disease that aggressively attacks the liver and digestive tract. In mild cases, the symptoms are similar to the flu and are often misdiagnosed, but, in serious cases, known as the toxic phase, the patient develops a high temperature and then encounters a series of life-threatening conditions such as internal bleeding, kidney failure, liver failure, and meningitis.

In the early stages, yellow fever is sometimes difficult to detect, since symptoms overlap with those associated with malaria, typhoid, hepatitis, and poisoning of various kinds, but, in its toxic phase—the mortality rate for patients in the toxic phase is around 50 percent—patients develop jaundice caused by liver failure, and they spew large quantities of so-called black vomit.

Symptoms appear from one to six days after infection. Typically, the disease will go through three stages. In the first stage, the patient will experience a high fever, headaches, and a rapid pulse. Later, the patient's pulse will fall below normal, and he will experience pains in the limbs and back. The second stage brings relief from the symptoms of the first stage and creates a false sense of security. In the third stage, the disease escalates, and the patient experiences jaundice and vomits black blood. At that stage, death usually follows within ten to fourteen days.

Yellow fever is transmitted by the *Aedes aegypti* mosquito, indigenous to most parts, but some researchers believe that it can be spread by close personal contact with infected persons if there is needle sharing or contact with blood during sexual intercourse. A mosquito can pick up the virus if it bites an infected person, but it must incubate for at least eight days inside the mosquito before the insect can give the disease to another human. After twelve days, the mosquito can transmit the disease for as long as it lives. It only takes a handful of infected mosquitoes to instigate an epidemic. That's because noninfected mosquitoes can become infected simply by biting an infected person.

There are three types of transmission cycles for yellow fever:

- *Sylvatic (or jungle) yellow fever*: Monkeys become infected by mosquitoes in tropical rainforests and then pass the virus on to other mosquitoes that feed on them. Humans that enter that jungle environment become infected after being bitten by the infected mosquitoes. Most of the people who acquire this type of yellow fever are young men who enter the jungle to work for logging or mining operations.

- *Intermediate yellow fever:* This particular strain is found only in the humid or semi-humid savannahs of Africa. Typically, many separate villages experience outbreaks simultaneously and then spread the disease to more populated areas as the human-monkey-mosquito cycle expands its reach.
- *Urban yellow fever:* This mode of transmission occurs when migrants introduce the disease into areas of high human population density. Unlike intermediate yellow fever, monkeys are not involved in the transmission of the disease. It is confined to humans and mosquitoes.[8]

Dr. Hayes feels that there is a need for American physicians to be better educated about the symptoms and treatment for yellow fever. "Because of air traffic, it is possible for someone to go to the Amazon region of Brazil or Columbia, and come back with yellow fever," he says.[9] "That person may come into a place that is relatively inexperienced as far as the medical staff is concerned, especially if they are not accustomed to dealing with tropical diseases. It's very important that in the global situation that we live in that doctors have an understanding of diseases that they might otherwise consider too exotic for them to ever see, and it is important for doctors to understand the importance of reporting any cases of yellow fever to their health departments, so that the epidemiological response can be appropriately initiated to make sure that there will not be endemic transmission should a mosquito bite the patient."

Hayes is confident that the CDC would be able to handle a yellow fever outbreak in a large city such as Miami. "I think we would be able to control it," he says, "but the other problem is the public reaction to the situation and the high demand for vaccine. If the entire city of Miami said it wanted to get vaccinated, then we might have a vaccine supply problem. Why? Because the regulation in the U.S. for which vaccines you can administer are more stringent [than in other countries]."

Aside from the fallout of a yellow fever terrorist attack, the CDC's greatest concern is over an outbreak in South America. "That is the most likely scenario, the one with which we are quite concerned," says Hayes. "There are heavy infestations of mosquitoes in those heavily populated cities where people are living without protection from mosquitoes. If [an infected person] came back into an urban area and started a cycle of urban yellow fever, we really would have a problem on our hands. Given our current vaccine protection, probably within a few days we would be able to mobilize most of the doses necessary to deal with that situation and then try to prompt rapid production of additional doses; but that would have to be done by eliciting the cooperation of the various yellow fever production companies in various countries, such as Brazil and England."

There is no cure for yellow fever, nor is there a treatment specific to the disease. Physicians typically treat the symptoms, doing what they can to alleviate pain, control vomiting, and correct dehydration and fever. It also is important to control any internal bleeding that occurs. In some cases, antibiotics are used to combat accompanying bacterial infections, but good judgment must be used in choosing antibiotics that do not cause liver or kidney failure as a side effect.[10]

ONE LAST FRIGHTENING LOOK AT THE RAVAGES OF YELLOW FEVER

It is one thing to read about the symptoms of yellow fever—they are frightening, to be sure—but it is another thing to read about what happens inside your body once the disease has run its course and left you a corpse. For that type of understanding, the only appropriate guide is an autopsy report. What follows is the 1925 autopsy report of a yellow fever victim by the name of Robert Sherman, an engineer from Nevada:

First, the physician who performed the autopsy, Dr. G. Jameson Carr, noted that the bed on which the body lay was stained in the center with a large, dark-brown patch that was intermingled with a few splotches of bright red blood and urine that was passed at the time of death. He noted an odor of urine. Carr also noted that he had a complete double set of gold crowns in his mouth and an old healed scar on his left hand. There was a scar from and old healed ulcer in the upper third of the external surface of the penis and an old tattoo of an American flag over an American eagle.

Carr's report continues verbatim:

Appearance of the Body—The body shows marked post-mortem lividity, especially in the dependent parts with marked congestion of the face and upper chest, the whole body being of a dirty ochre yellow color, most marked in the conjunctiva, face, upper chest and both sides of the abdomen, but particularly marked around the region of the genitalia and the anterior upper third of the thighs. There is oozing of a brown fluid from the mouth and from the rectum a considerable quantity of this brown fluid, but mixed with bright red blood. The mouth and posterior nasal passage contains a brown fluid.

Heart—In the state of diastole, the right heart containing post mortem fluid blood. The myocardium was yellowish and of a dull luster but no eccymosis were seen. The endocardium, especially the papillary muscles were distinctly yellow. There was a healed sortitis of the first part of the aorta with calcareous plaques and calcareous resolution of vegetations on the aorta.

Liver—The liver was enlarged. The surface had marked yellow and bluish mottling of fine design. On section very friable and a uniform dirty yellow.

Gastro-Intestinal System—The stomach and intestines were involved in an enormous mass of bright yellow fat. The stomach itself contained a dark green content, the serosa appeared normal, the sub-mucosa was of a chocolate color while the mucosa was minutely and intensely injected with ecchymosis at the cardiac end. The small intestines contained a similar fluid while the colon contents were more tarry in nature.

Kidneys—The kidneys were enlarged hyperaemic and of a yellowish brown color. Owning to the enormously thick capsule of fat, firmly adherent to the true capsule of the kidney it was shelled out entire and with ease. One section, marked hyperrhaemia of the cortex especially at the junction of the cortex and medulla, while the medulla itself was stained yellow and in the pelvis was a mass of bright yellow fat.

WHAT YOU SHOULD KNOW ABOUT THE YELLOW FEVER VACCINE

The best protection against yellow fever is vaccination. Immunity occurs within one week in 95 percent of the people vaccinated and provides protection for a minimum of ten years and possibly for life. Over 300 million doses have been given, with only moderate side effects, but, for reasons not understood by researchers, there have been a series of unexplained deaths as a result of the vaccination in several countries, including Brazil, Australia, and the United States, where the vaccine is available only to people traveling to infected areas.

"There is this concern that it is not good to die from a vaccine, so we are trying to figure out why and look at risk factors for this problem and to better understand the immune response following the vaccine," says Hayes.[11] "Any residents of the U.S. who are traveling to an area where yellow fever is being transmitted would be recommended to get the vaccine. The problem seems to be particularly in people over sixty years of age. The risk is less than four per 100,000, but the risk of getting yellow fever is quite low for a tourist going to an endemic area for a short period. You have very low, but competing risks, so for older individuals the question of getting vaccinated has become more problematic. We are trying to figure out why this is happening. We don't have evidence that the vaccine has changed. We think it is more related to people's genetics, or host responses to people that get the vaccine."

Vaccination against yellow fever is recommended for all persons nine months of age and older who travel to or live in areas where the disease is active and for anyone who might come into contact with the virus. If you are in either of these categories, you should consider the following:

- The vaccine available in the United States and Canada is grown in chicken embryo cells and will likely contain egg or chicken protein. If you are allergic to eggs or chicken, you should ask your physician to perform a skin allergy test before taking the vaccine. If you need the vaccine to travel to a country that requires a vaccination certificate, then you should ask your physician to write you a letter requesting a waiver because of your allergies.
- Side effects to the vaccine are rare, but they must be factored into your decision, especially if you are over sixty. An increasing number of individuals are dying from reactions to the vaccine for reasons unknown. Other serious side effects include confusion, convulsions, difficulty breathing or swallowing, severe headaches, throbbing in the ears, fast heartbeat, and vomiting.
- Drug reactions should be considered, so please advise your physician of all prescription drugs you are taking. Also advise your physician if you are being treated for organ transplants or cancer, since x-rays and some medicines may decrease the useful effect of the vaccine and may increase the possibility of side effects.

- Yellow fever vaccine can cause birth defects, so it is not recommended for pregnant women unless they are at high risk of getting the disease.

Like a dark and stormy cloud, yellow fever hovers in South America, slowly being drawn north to the United States by the effects of global warming. Even more ominously, it has the potential of being used in America as a weapon of mass destruction by impatient terrorists unwilling to allow nature to take its course. America's survival as a nation, at some point in the not too distant future, may depend on its understanding of its worst enemy, *yellow fever*.

SYMPTOMS OF YELLOW FEVER

EARLY PHASE
Fever
Headache
Backache
Shivers
Loss of appetite

TOXIC PHASE
Abdominal pain
Jaundice
Bleeding from mouth, nose, eyes, or stomach
"Black" vomit (caused by stomach bleeding)
Kidney failure (no urine production)
Liver failure (basically the same symptoms as liver cancer)

There is a 50 percent mortality rate for patients who enter the toxic phase.

HOW TO PROTECT YOURSELF
AGAINST YELLOW FEVER

- Vaccination (if over 60, discuss severity of the threat with a physician).
- If traveling abroad, be alert to reports of yellow fever outbreaks. Because of the way the disease is transmitted, one case is considered an outbreak.
- Apply insect repellent to exposed skin. DEET is toxic if swallowed, so do not breathe in, swallow, or get into the eyes. If applying DEET to your face, spray your hands and rub the product carefully over the face, avoiding eyes and mouth. Children under 10 should not apply insect repellent themselves.
- Wear long-sleeved shirts, long pants, and hats. Protect infants by using a carrier draped with mosquito netting with an elastic edge for a tight fit.
- Pay special attention to the threat of mosquito bites between dusk and dawn, for that is when mosquitoes are most active.

notes

CHAPTER ONE

1. J. Worth Estes and Billy G. Smith, *Old Family Letters Relating to the Yellow Fever* (Philadelphia: J. B. Lippincott, 1892); Estes and Smith, *A Melancholy Scene of Devastation* (Philadelphia: Science History Publications, 1997).

2. Mathew Carey, *A Short Account of the Malignant Fever, Lately Prevalent in Philadelphia* (Philadelphia: Mathew Carey, 1794).

3. Estes and Smith, *Melancholy Scene of Devastation.*

4. J. H. Powell, *Bring Out Your Dead* (Philadelphia: University of Pennsylvania Press, 1949).

5. Ibid.

6. Jim Murphy, *An American Plague* (New York: Clarion Books, 2003).

7. Helen Bryan, *Martha Washington: First Lady of Liberty* (New York: John Wiley & Sons, 2002).

8. John R. Pierce and Jim Writer, *Yellow Jack* (Hoboken, NJ: John Wiley & Sons, 2005).

9. Powell, *Bring Out Your Dead.*

10. Murphy, *American Plague.*

11. Powell, *Bring Out Your Dead.*

12. Bryan, *Martha Washington.*

CHAPTER TWO

1. Willard Sterne Randall, *Thomas Jefferson: A Life* (New York: Henry Holt, 1993).

2. Jim Fraiser and West Freeman, *The French Quarter of New Orleans* (Jackson: University Press of Mississippi, 2003).

3. John Duffy, *Sword of Pestilence* (Baton Rouge: Louisiana State University Press, 1966).

4. Peter Finney Jr., "West Nile Epidemic Recalls Yellow Fever," *Clarion Herald*, August 14, 2002.

5. *Daily Delta*, July 17, 1853.

6. *Daily Delta,* September 4, 1853.

7. Geoffrey C. Ward and Ken Burns, *Jazz: A History of America's Music* (New York: Alfred A. Knopf, 2000).

8. Margaret Humphreys, *Yellow Fever and the South* (Baltimore: Johns Hopkins University Press, 1992).

9. John H. Ellis, *Yellow Fever & Public Health in the New South* (Lexington: University Press of Kentucky, 1992).

10. Khaled J. Bloom, *The Mississippi Valley's Great Yellow Fever Epidemic of 1878* (Baton Rouge: Louisiana State University Press, 1993).

11. *New York Times*, September 3, 1878.

12. *New Orleans Picayune*, September 11, 1878.

13. *New Orleans Picayune*, November 1, 1878.

CHAPTER THREE

1. One of the fort's commanders was a lieutenant named Zachary Taylor, who later became America's twelfth president.

2. *Los Angeles Times*, 1999.

3. John E. Harkins, *Metropolis of the American Nile* (Woodland Hills, CA: Windsor Publications, 1982).

4. Ibid.

5. *In Memoriam of the Lamented Dead Who Fell in Memphis during the Yellow Fever Epidemic* (Memphis: Southern Publishing, 1874).

6. *Memphis Appeal,* September 7, 1873.

7. Rev. D. A. Quin, *Heroes and Heroines of Memphis; or Reminiscences of the Yellow Fever Epidemic That Afflicted the City of Memphis during the Autumn Months of 1873, 1878, and 1879* (Providence, RI: E. L. Freeman & Son, 1874).

8. Belle Wade's diary is part of the yellow fever collection in the Memphis Room of the Memphis and Shelby County Public Library.

9. *Memphis Avalanche*, August 9–10, 1878.

10. *Southern Jewish Heritage* 15, no. 1 (Spring 2002).

11. *Memphis Avalanche*, August 27, 1878.

12. Dr. J. P. Dromgoole, *Yellow Fever: Heroes, Honors, and Horrors* (Louisville, KY: John P. Morton, 1879).

13. Walter Stewart, "Bring Out Your Dead," *Memphis Press-Scimitar*, April 7, 1932.

14. Van Dyke Collection, Mississippi Valley Collection, University of Memphis, Memphis, Tennessee.

15. Pamphlet printed in 1879, but not published.

16. Dromgoole, *Yellow Fever: Heroes, Honors, and Horrors.*

17. *Chicago Tribune*, September 24, 1878.

18. John H. Ellis, *Yellow Fever & Public Health in the New South* (Lexington: University Press of Kentucky, 1992).

19. Dromgoole, *Yellow Fever: Heroes, Honors and Horrors.*

20. *Memphis Appeal,* September 23, 1878.

CHAPTER FOUR

1. Dunbar Rowland, ed., *The Mississippi Territorial Archives, 1798–1803* (Nashville: Brandon Printing, 1905).

2. Christian Schultz, *Travels on an Inland Voyage* (New York: Isaac Riley, 1810).

3. Andrew R. Kilpatrick, "An Account of the Yellow Fever Which Prevailed in Woodville, Mississippi in the Year 1844," *New Orleans Medical Journal* (no publishing details available).

4. Ibid.

5. Montgomery County Historical Society.

6. Charles Manfred Thompson, *History of the United States* (Chicago: Benjamin H. Sanborn, 1927).

7. Edward S. Gregory. His comments can be found in *The Civil War: The American Iliad*, by Otto Eisenschiml and Ralph Newman.

8. Ibid.

9. Mississippi Department of Archives and History.

10. Deanne Nuwer, *The 1878 Yellow Fever Epidemic in Mississippi*, PhD diss., University of Southern Mississippi, 1996.

11. *Vicksburg Evening Post*, April 13, 1959.

12. Sister Mary Paulinus Oakes, *Angels of Mercy: An Eyewitness Account of Civil War and Yellow Fever* (Baltimore: Cathedral Foundation Press, 1998).

13. Nuwer, *1878 Yellow Fever Epidemic in Mississippi*.

14. Ibid.

15. J. L. Power, *Epidemic of 1878 in Mississippi* (Jackson, MS: Clarion Steam, 1879).

16. Susan Dabney Smedes, *Memorials of a Southern Planter* (Jackson: University Press of Mississippi, 1981).

17. Power, *Epidemic of 1878 in Mississippi*.

18. Mississippi Department of Archives and History.

19. Khaled J. Bloom, *The Mississippi Valley's Great Yellow Fever Epidemic of 1878* (Baton Rouge: Louisiana State University Press, 1993).

20. Dr. J. P. Dromgoole, *Yellow Fever: Heroes, Honors, and Horrors* (Louisville, KY: John P. Morton, 1879).

21. *New Orleans Picayune*, August 15, 1878.

22. Louise Meek, "Local Yellow Fever Epidemic Remembered by Grenadians," *Sentinel Star*, November 20, 1984.

23. Dromgoole, *Yellow Fever: Heroes, Honors, and Horrors*.

24. Nuwer, *1878 Yellow Fever Epidemic in Mississippi*.

25. Bob Lord, Washington County Historical Society, May 27, 1979.

26. Joseph T. Reily, Washington County Historical Society, December 7, 1980.

27. Ibid.

28. Bloom, *Mississippi Valley's Great Yellow Fever Epidemic of 1878*.

29. Dromgoole, *Yellow Fever: Heroes, Honors, and Horrors*.

30. *Vicksburg Evening Post*, May 4, 1983.

31. *Daily Bulletin*, September 22, 1897.

32. Mississippi Department of Archives and History.

CHAPTER FIVE

1. Charles Morrow Wilson, *Ambassadors in White* (Port Washington, NY: Kennikat Press, 1972).

2. François Delaporte, *The History of Yellow Fever: An Essay on the Birth of Tropical Medicine* (Cambridge, MA: MIT Press, 1991).

3. William B. Bean, *Walter Reed: A Biography* (Charlottesville: University Press of Virginia, 1982).

4. Ibid.

5. Ibid.

6. *New York Times,* February 15, 1898.

7. Theophilus G. Steward, *The Colored Regulars in the United States Army* (Philadelphia: A.M.E. Book Concern, 1904).

8. Wilson, *Ambassadors in White.*

9. Dianne Greenhill, "Lena Angevine Warner: Pioneer Public Health Nurse," *Public Health Nursing* 11, no. 3 (1994): 202–204.

10. Bean, *Walter Reed: A Biography.*

11. Ibid.

12. Greenhill, "Lena Angevine Warner."

13. *Chicago Record*, 1900, Philip S. Hench Walter Reed Yellow Fever Collection.

14. *New York Times*, October 27, 1900, Philip S. Hench Walter Reed Yellow Fever Collection.

15. Bean, *Walter Reed: A Biography.*

16. "How Yellow Fever Was Conquered," *American Association for Medical Progress* [undated], Philip S. Hench Walter Reed Yellow Fever Collection.

17. Letter from Walter Reed to Emilie Reed [undated], Philip S. Hench Walter Reed Yellow Fever Collection.

18. Letter from Walter Reed to Laura Reed Blincoe, March 26, 1901, Philip S. Hench Walter Reed Yellow Fever Collection.

19. "What Surgeon General Sternberg Says," *Washington Post,* April 19, 1901.

20. *Times of Cuba*, March 1918, reprinted March 23, 1918, by the *New York Tribune*, Philip S. Hench Walter Reed Yellow Fever Collection.

21. Bob Cullen, "A Man, A Plan, A Canal: Panama Rises," *Smithsonian* (March 2004).

22. Wilson, *Ambassadors in White.*

23. Ibid.

24. Charles S. Bryan, *Most Satisfactory Man: The Story of Theodore Brevard Hayne, Last Martyr of Yellow Fever* (Spartanburg, SC: Reprint, 1996).

CHAPTER SIX

1. Frank Prentice Rand, *The Village of Amherst: A Landmark of Light* (Amherst, MA: Amherst Historical Society, 1958).

2. Major Charles E. Heller, "Chemical Warfare in World War I: The American Experience, 1917–1918," *Combat Studies Institute, U.S. Army Command and General Staff College* (September 1984): 6–7.

3. Augustin M. Prentiss, *Chemicals in War: A Treatise on Chemical Warfare* (New York: McGraw-Hill, 1937).

4. Heller, "Chemical Warfare in World War I."

5. S. H. Harris, *Factories of Death: Japanese Biological Warfare, 1932–45, and the American Cover-Up* (New York: Routledge, 1994).

6. L. B. Seeff, G. W. Beebe, and J. H. Hoofnagle et al., "A Serologic Follow-Up of the 1942 Epidemic of Post-Vaccination Hepatitis in the United States Army," *New England Medical Journal* 316, no. 16 (April 187): 965–70.

7. Martin Furmanski, "Unlicensed Vaccines and Bioweapon Defense in World War II," originally published in the *Journal of the American Medical Association*, it was subsequently made available at www.gulfwarvets.com.

8. J. Perry Robinson, "Chemical Weapons," in *CBW: Chemical and Biological Warfare*, ed. Steven Rose (Boston: Beacon Press, 1968).

9. Catholicexchange.com, posted March 20, 2002.

10. Edward M. Eitzen and Ernest T. Takafuji, "Historical Overview of Biological Warfare," *Virtual Naval Hospital*, 1997, 2005.

11. Judith Miller, Stephen Engelberg, and William Broad, *Germs: Biological Weapons and America's Secret War* (New York: Simon & Schuster, 2002).

12. Interview with Bill Patrick for *NOVA* in 2001. The interview was conducted by *NOVA* producer Kirk Wolfinger and *New York Times* reporter Bill Broad.

13. Author interview, March 3, 2005.

14. Miller, Engelberg, and Broad, *Germs: Biological Weapons and America's Secret War.*

15. Steven Rose, ed., *CBW: Chemical and Biological Warfare* (Boston: Beacon Press, 1968).

16. Thomas W. McGovern and Chad Hivnor, "Dermatologic Aspects of Bioterrorism Agents," Emedicine.com (updated June 29, 2004).

17. *NOVA* interview.

18. BBC interview broadcast on March 14, 2002, on the program *Newsnight.*

19. Commodity Research Bureau.

20. Author interview.

21. McGovern and Hivnor, "Dermatologic Aspects of Bioterrorism Agents."

22. L. Borio, T. Inglesby, C. J. Peters et al., "Hemorrhagic Fever *Viruses* as Biological Weapons," *Journal of the American Medical Association* 287 (2002): 2391–405.

CHAPTER SEVEN

1. National Research Council, *Climate Change Science: An Analysis of Some Key Questions* (Washington, DC: National Academies Press, 2001).

2. James Gustave Speth, *Red Sky at Morning: America and the Crisis of the Global Environment* (New Haven, CT: Yale University Press, 2004).

3. National Research Council, *Climate Change Science.*

4. Ibid.

5. Richard W. Stevenson, "Bush Arrives at Summit Session, Ready to Stand Alone," *New York Times,* July 7, 2005.

6. Cat Lazaroff, "Warming Climate Spawns Disease Epidemics," *Environment News Service,* June 25, 2002. The study authored by Drew Harvell and Richard Ostfeld was originally published in the journal *Science* (June 21, 2002).

7. Author interview with Dr. Ned Hayes.

8. National Institute of Environmental Health Services, press release, March 9, 1998.

9. Paul R. Epstein, "Is Global Warming Harmful to Health?" *Scientific American* (August 20, 2000): 36–43.

10. Interview with Dr. Ned Hayes.

11. According to the CDC, as of July 2, 2005, early in the mosquito season, West Nile virus had been detected in Alabama, Arkansas, Arizona, California, Florida, Georgia, Iowa, Illinois, Indiana, Louisiana, Michigan, Minnesota, Missouri, Mississippi, New Jersey, New Mexico, New York, Ohio, Oklahoma, South Dakota, Tennessee, Texas, Wisconsin, and Wyoming.

12. Ibid.

CHAPTER EIGHT

1. A CNN news report based on a story released by the Environment News Network.

2. Information about Tom McCullough's death from yellow fever was published in an April 19, 2002, "Morbidity and Mortality Weekly Report" published by the Centers for Disease Control and Prevention, and from a March 27, 2002, story in the *Corpus Christi Caller-Times*, by Joy Victory.

3. "Morbidity and Mortality Weekly Report: Centers for Disease Control and Prevention," *Journal of the American Medical Association* 283, no. 17 (May 3, 2000).

4. Pedro F. C. Vasconcelos, Juliet E. Bryant, T. P. da Rosa, Robert B. Tesh, Sueli G. Rodrigues, and Alan D. T. Barrett, "Genetic Divergence and Dispersal of Yellow Fever Virus, Brazil," *Emerging Infectious Diseases* 10, no. 9 (September 2004): 1578–84.

5. Fred L. Soper, "The Newer Epidemiology of Yellow Fever," *American Journal of Public Health* (January 1937).

6. Ibid.

7. Author interview.

8. World Health Organization.

9. Author interview

10. United States Centers for Disease Control and Prevention and World Health Organization.

11. Author interview.

bibliography

BOOKS

Athanasiou, Tom, and Paul Baer. *Dead Heat: Global Justice and Global Warming*. New York: Seven Stories, 2002.

Bean, William B. *Walter Reed: A Biography*. Charlottesville: University Press of Virginia, 1982.

Bloom, Khaled J. *The Mississippi Valley's Great Yellow Fever Epidemic of 1878*. Baton Rouge: Louisiana State University Press, 1993.

Bryan, Charles S. *A Most Satisfactory Man: The Story of Theodore Brevard Hayne, Last Martyr of Yellow Fever*. Spartanburg, SC: Reprint, 1996.

Bryan, Helen. *Martha Washington: First Lady of Liberty*. New York: John Wiley & Sons, 2002.

Carey, Mathew. *A Short Account of the Malignant Fever, Lately Prevalent in Philadelphia*. Philadelphia: Mathew Carey, 1794.

Delaporte, François. *The History of Yellow Fever: An Essay on the Birth of Tropical Medicine*. Cambridge, MA: MIT Press, 1991.

Dromgoole, Dr. J. P. *Yellow Fever: Heroes, Honors, and Horrors*. Louisville, KY: John P. Morton, 1879.

Duffy, John. *Sword of Pestilence*. Baton Rouge: Louisiana State University Press, 1966.

Eisenschiml, Otto, and Ralph Newman. *The Civil War: The American Iliad*. Vol. 1. New York: Grosset & Dunlap, 1956.

Ellis, John H. *Yellow Fever & Public Health in the New South*. Lexington: University Press of Kentucky, 1992.

Estes, J. Worth, and Billy G. Smith. *Old Family Letters Relating to the Yellow Fever.* Philadelphia: J. B. Lippincott, 1892.

——. *A Melancholy Scene of Devastation.* Canton, MA: Science History Publications, 1997.

Fraiser, Jim, and West Freeman. *The French Quarter of New Orleans.* Jackson: University Press of Mississippi, 2003.

Grant, Ulysses S. *The Civil War Memoirs of Ulysses S. Grant.* Abridged edition edited by Thomas Fleming. New York: Tom Doherty, 2002.

Harkins, John E. *Metropolis of the American Nile: An Illustrated History of Memphis and Shelby County.* Woodland Hills, CA: Windsor Publications, 1982.

Harris, S. H. *Factories of Death: Japanese Biological Warfare, 1932–45, and the American Cover-Up.* New York: Routledge, 1994.

Henry, R. H. *Editors I Have Known since the Civil War.* Jackson, MS: R. H. Henry, 1922.

Howard, Hugh. *Natchez: The Houses and History of the Jewel of the Mississippi.* New York: Rizzoli, 2003.

Humphreys, Margaret. *Yellow Fever and the South.* Baltimore: Johns Hopkins University Press, 1992.

Keating, J. M. *The Yellow Fever Epidemic of 1878 in Memphis, Tenn.* Memphis: Howard Association, 1879.

LaPointe, Patricia. *From Saddlebags to Science: A Century of Health Care in Memphis, 1830–1930.* Memphis: Health Sciences Museum Foundation of the Memphis and Shelby County Medical Society Auxiliary, 1984.

Miller, Judith, Stephen Engelberg, and William Broad. *Germs: Biological Weapons and America's Secret War.* New York: Simon & Schuster, 2002.

Murphy, Jim. *An American Plague.* New York: Clarion Books, 2003.

National Research Council. *Chemical and Biological Terrorism: Research and Development to Improve Civilian Medical Response.* Washington, DC: National Academy Press, 1999.

——. *Climate Change Science: An Analysis of Some Key Questions.* Washington, DC: National Academy Press, 2001.

Oakes, Sister Mary Paulinus. *Angels of Mercy: An Eyewitness Account of Civil War and Yellow Fever.* Baltimore: Cathedral Foundation Press, 1998.

Pierce, John R., and Jim Writer. *Yellow Jack.* Hoboken, NJ: John Wiley & Sons, 2005.

Polk, Noel, ed. *Natchez before 1830*. Jackson: University Press of Mississippi, 1989.

Powell, J. H. *Bring Out Your Dead: The Great Plague of Yellow Fever in Philadelphia in 1793*. Philadelphia: University of Pennsylvania Press, 1949. Reprint, New York: Time Reading Program, 1965.

Power, J. L. *Epidemic of 1878 in Mississippi*. Jackson, MS: Clarion Steam, 1879.

Prentiss, Augustin M. *Chemicals in War: A Treatise on Chemical Warfare*. New York: McGraw-Hill, 1937.

Quin, Rev. D. A. *Heroes and Heroines of Memphis; or Reminiscences of the Yellow Fever Epidemics That Afflicted the City of Memphis during the Autumn Months of 1873, 1878, and 1879*. Providence, RI: E. L. Freeman & Son, 1874.

Rand, Frank Prentice. *The Village of Amherst: A Landmark of Light*. Amherst, MA: Amherst Historical Society, 1958.

Randall, J. G., and David Donald. *The Civil War and Reconstruction*. Lexington, MA: D. C. Heath, 1969.

Randall, Willard Sterne. *Thomas Jefferson: A Life*. New York: Henry Holt, 1993.

Robinson, J. Perry. "Chemical Weapons." In *CBW: Chemical and Biological Warfare*, edited by Steven Rose. Boston: Beacon Press, 1968.

Rowland, Dunbar, ed. *The Mississippi Territorial Archives, 1798–1803*. Nashville: Brandon Printing, 1905.

Rose, Steven, ed. *CBW: Chemical and Biological Warfare*. Boston: Beacon Press, 1968.

Sanford, William R. *The Natchez Trace Historic Trail in American History*. Berkeley Heights, NJ: Enslow, 2001.

Schultz, Christian. *Travels on an Inland Voyage*. New York: Isaac Riley, 1810.

Smedes, Susan Dabney. *Memorials of a Southern Planter*. Jackson: University Press of Mississippi, 1981.

Speth, James Gustave. *Red Sky at Morning: America and the Crisis of the Global Environment*. New Haven, CT: Yale University Press, 2004.

Steward, Theophilus G. *Colored Regulars in the United States Army*. Philadelphia: A.M.E. Book Concern, 1904.

Thompson, Charles Manfred. *History of the United States*. Chicago: Benjamin H. Sanborn, 1922.

Ward, Geoffrey C., with Ken Burns. *Jazz: A History of America's Music.* New York: Alfred A. Knopf, 2000.

Wiencek, Henry. *An Imperfect God: George Washington, His Slaves, and the Creation of America.* New York: Farrar, Straus and Giroux, 2003.

Wills, Christopher. *Yellow Fever, Black Goddess: The Coevolution of People and Plagues.* Reading, MA: Addison-Wesley, 1996.

Wilson, Charles Morrow. *Ambassadors in White.* Port Washington, NY: Kennikat Press, 1972.

PERIODICALS

Borio, L., T. Inglesby, C. J. Peters et al. "Hemorrhagic Fever *Viruses* as Biological Weapons." *Journal of the American Medical Association* 287 (2002): 2391–405.

Cullen, Bob. "A Man, A Plan, A Canal: Panama Rises." *Smithsonian* (March 2004).

Eitzen, Edward M. and Ernest T. Takafuji. "Historical Overview of Biological Warfare." *Virtual Naval Hospital,* http://www.vnh.org, 1997, 2005.

Epstein, Paul R. "Is Global Warming Harmful to Health?" *Scientific American* (August 20, 2000): 36–43.

Finney, Peter, Jr. "West Nile Epidemic Recalls Yellow Fever." *Clarion Herald,* August 14, 2002.

Furman, Bess. "Fever of Jungle Marching North." *New York Times,* February 12, 1956.

Furmanski, Martin. "Unlicensed Vaccines and Bioweapon Defense in World War II." Originally published in the *Journal of the American Medical Association,* it was subsequently made available at www.gulfwarvets.com.

Greenhill, Dianne. "Lena Angevine Warner: Pioneer Public Health Nurse." *Public Health Nursing* 11, no. 3 (1994): 202–204.

Heller, Major Charles E. "Chemical Warfare in World War I: The American Experience, 1917–1918." *Combat Studies Institute, U.S. Army Command and General Staff College* (September 1984): 6–7.

Kilpatrick, Andrew R. "An Account of the Yellow Fever Which prevailed in Woodville, Mississippi in the Year 1844." *New Orleans Medical Journal.* [No publishing details available.]

Landhuis, Esther. "Scientists Pursue West Nile Vaccine." *San Jose Mercury News*, October 4, 2003.

Lazaroff, Cat. "Warming Climate Spawns Disease Epidemics." *Environment News Service*, June 25, 2002. The study authored by Drew Harvell and Richard Ostfeld was originally published in the journal *Science*, June 21, 2002.

McFarland, Patricia LaPointe. "Yellow Fever: The 'King of Terrors'/The Memphis Jewish Community in the Epidemic of 1878." *Southern Jewish Heritage* (Spring 2002).

Meek, Louise. "Local Yellow Fever Epidemic Remembered by Grenadians." *Grenada (Mississippi) Sentinel Star,* November 20, 1984.

Pantenburg, Leon. "Yankee Was Hero in City's Battle with Yellow Fever." *Vicksburg (Mississippi) Post*, October 26, 1983.

Reed, Walter. "The Etiology of Yellow Fever—An Additional Note." Presented February 6, 1901, at a meeting of the American Public Health Association.

Sawyer, W. A., W. D. M. Lloyd, and S. F. Kitchen. "The Rockefeller Foundation." Published by the International Health Division of the Rockefeller Foundation and the Rockefeller Institute for Medical Research (March 28, 1929).

Seeff, L. B., G. W. Beebe, J. H. Hoofnagle, J. E. Norman, Z. Buskell-Bales, J. G. Waggoner, N. Kaplowitz, R. S. Koff, J. L. Petrini Jr., and E. R. Schiff. "A Serologic Follow-Up of the 1942 Epidemic of Post-Vaccination Hepatitis in the United States Army." *New England Medical Journal* 316, no. 16 (April 1987): 965–70.

Shaw, Jonathan. "Battling Bioterrorism." *Harvard Magazine* 104 (January–February 2002).

Sisler, George. "The Time Memphis Died." *Commercial Appeal*, August 24, 1958.

Soper, Fred L. "The Newer Epidemiology of Yellow Fever." *American Journal of Public Health*, January 1937.

Stevenson, Richard W. "Bush Arrives at Summit Session, Ready to Stand Alone." *New York Times*, July 7, 2005.

Stewart, Walter. "Bring Out Your Dead." *Memphis Press-Scimitar*, April 7, 1932.

Vasconcelos, Pedro F. C., Juliet E. Bryant, T. P. da Rosa, Robert B. Tesh, Sueli G. Rodrigues, and Alan D. T. Barrett. "Genetic Divergence and

Dispersal of Yellow Fever Virus, Brazil." *Emerging Infectious Diseases* 10, no. 9 (September 2004): 1578–84 .

Victory, Joy. "CDC Confirms Local Man Died of Yellow Fever." *Corpus Christi Caller-Times*, March 27, 2002.

———. "Local Man Dies after a Fishing Trip to Brazil." *Corpus Christi Caller-Times*, March 19, 2002.

Wilemon, Tom. "Yellow Fever Struck Home." *Daily Corinthian*, April 25, 1995.

ELECTRONIC MEDIA

Broad, Bill, and Kirk Wolfinger. "Interviews with Biowarriors." BBC.com (updated November 2001).

McGovern, Thomas W., and George W. Christopher. "Biological Warfare and Its Cutaneous Manifestations." Telemedicine.org.

McGovern, Thomas W., and Chad Hivnor. "Dermatologic Aspects of Bioterrorism Agents." Emedicine.com. Last updated June 29, 2004.

index

Adams, John, 17; letter from Benjamin Rush, 15
Amherst, Lord Jeffrey, 187
anthrax, 209, 219–20
Archer, Stevenson, 135
Augusta, 40–41

Bee, 69
Bell, Dr. A. N., 173
Ben Allen, 134
biological warfare, history of, 187–88; World War I, 188–90; yellow fever, 199–200; use in Vietnam, 203, 205–206; Islamic mindset, 210–12, 216
Bionda, Kate, 78
botulism, 220–21
Bradbury, John, 62–63
bubonic plague, 224
Buford, Mary, 121
Burleigh Plantation, 123
Bush, President George W., 208–209, 228; rejects Kyoto Protocol, 229; rejects Group of 8 position on global warming, 239
Butler, General Benjamin, 49

Camboden Castle, 40
Camp Detrick (Fort Detrick), 195–96, 199; testing in Mississippi, 201–202, 207, 209–10
Carey, Mathew, 25–26
Carr, Dr. G. Jameson, 247
Carroll, Dr. James, 163; death of, 165, 166–78
Catholic Sisters of Mercy, 119–20
Charlie B. Woods, 54
Cherbin, Dr. Nicholas, 37
Chief Pushmataha, 105
Choppin, Samuel, 52
Civil War, population, 113–14; reconstruction, 116
Clairborne, William, 106–108
Clapp, Theodore, 37, 43–44
Clark, William, 61
Clarkson, Mayor Matthew, 19, 26
Cook, Annie, 82–83

Creoles, origins of, 35
Crossman, Mayor A. D., 39
Currie, Dr. William, 16, 24

Dabney, Susan, 123–24
Dabney, Thomas, 123
Daltroff, Louis, 94
Davis, Dr. Charles T., 83
Davis, Jefferson, 69; death of son, 96; yellow fever epidemic, Rosemont Plantation, 109
Dobson, Andrew, 231–32
Dromgoole, Dr. J. P., 93–94; yellow fever in Greenville, Mississippi, 127

Ebola, 223
Emily B. Souder, 53–55
Epstein, Paul R., 231, 233–34

Falvo, Dr. Cathey, 236
Farragut, Admiral David, 49
Fenner, Dr. Erasmus Darwin, 40–41
Finley, Dr. Juan Carlos, background of, 141–42, 143–45, 153, 161
Forrest, General Nathan Bedford, 69
Fort Pickering, 61
Foulke, John, 14–15
Franklin, Benjamin, 27
French Quarter, location of, 35
Fulton City, 69–70

Geneva Protocol of 1925, 191
global warming, 225
Gorgas, Dr. William, 148–49, 163, 166–69, 172; illness of, 173; death of, 174, 175–77, 181–84
Grant, General Ulysses, 114, 116
Grenada, Mississippi, 77, 85, 126–27, 129, 133, 159, 265
Greenville, Mississippi, 132–35
Guiteras, Dr. Juan, 176–77

Hamilton, Alexander, 22, 29
Harper, Annie, 114
Harvell, Drew, 231
Hayes, Dr. Ned, 202–203; on yellow fever as biological weapon, 213, 216, 232, 234–35, 242–43, 246
Hayes, President Rutherford B., 52
Hearst, William Randolph, 150–51
Heler, Charles E., 188
Henner, Anna Marie, 137
Hersh, Seymour M., 203
Hitler, Adolf, 192
Hood, General John Bell, 137
Hussein, Saddam, 207

Intergovernmental Panel of Climate Change (IPCC), 226–27

Jackson, Andrew, 64–65
Jefferson, Thomas, 22, 30, 33; purchase of Louisiana Territory, 34, 61, 107
John M. Chambers, 93, 120
John Porter, 75, 117–18
Jones, Absalom, 26

Kate Dickson, 134
Kean, Jefferson Randolph, 159, 161

Keating, Dr. Michael, 93
Keller, Susan, 111
Kilpatrick, Dr. Andrew, 109–11
Kissinger, Henry, 204
Kissinger, John R., 168–69
Knox, Henry, 22

Latrobe, Benjamin Henry, 35–36
Lazear, Jesse, 159, 163–67
Lear, Tobins, 22
Lee, Thomas, 28–29
LeMaigre, Catherine, 14–15
LeMaigre, Peter, 14
Lewis, Colonel J. S., 109
Lewis, Meriwether, 61–62

MacArthur, General Douglas, 198;
    accused of using yellow fever
    in North Korea, 201
Madison, President James, 62
Manhattan Engineer District,
    196–97
McCullough, Stephanie, 238–39
McCullough, Tom, 237–40
McDowell, Katharine Bonnere,
    120–32
McGovern, Dr. Thomas, 206,
    214–15
McKinley, President William,
    149–50
Memphis, reconstruction, 68–69
Menken, Nathan, 79
Merck, George W., 195
Meselson, Matthew, 204
Mifflin, Thomas, 19, 30
Mississippi Delta, Indian culture,
    112, 113, 116

Mississippi Quarantine Station, 52
Mueller, Karl, 64

Nashville, Tennessee, 62, 68, 99–
    100, 107–108, 180, 255, 263
Natchez Indians, 103–104
Natchez, Mississippi, history of,
    103–104
Natchez Trace, 62, 106–107
New Madrid earthquakes, 63
New Orleans, first yellow fever epi-
    demic, 33; slave trade, 34, 36,
    38, 39, 40–42; grand jury
    report, 45, 46–48; civil war, 49,
    51; reconstruction, 50, 51–53,
    55–56, 58
Nixon, President Richard, ends
    offensive biological warfare
    program, 204–205

Oppenheimer, J. Robert, 197
Ostfeld, Richard, 231
Overton, Judge John, 64

Panama, yellow fever, 179–84;
    President Roosevelt visits, 183,
    241, 257, 264
Patrick, Bill, 201–202, 209–10, 214
Patz, Jonathan, 233
Pensacola, Florida, yellow fever
    epidemic of 1765, 108
Pickering, Timothy, 29, 61
Pine Bluff Arsenal, 201
Polk, General Leonidas, 66

Quin, Rev. S. A., 71

Raine, Julie, 125
Randolph, Edmund, 29
Raymond, W. C., 51
Reed, Emilee, 147, 174
Reed, Walter, background of, 145–48, 157–59, 161, 164–69, 172; illness of, 173; death of, 174
Richardson, Phoebe, 111
Rickover, Admiral Hyman G., 157
Roosevelt, President Franklin, 192–93
Roosevelt, Theodore, 154, 180
Rush, Dr. Benjamin, 14–20, 23–25, 29
Rush, Julia, 16, 25, 30

Sargent, Winthrop, 104–106
Sawyer, Dr. Wilbur, 185, 200
Schultz, Christian, 105–106
Schuppert, Dr. Moritz, 41–42
Shaw, Ed, 69
Sherman, General William, arrives at Fort Pickering, 67; invades Mississippi, 114
Sigsbee, Charles, 151
Silvers, Charley, 91
smallpox, 218–19
Soper, Dr. Fred L., 242
Speth, James Gustave, 227–28
Sternberg, Dr. George Miller, 142, 144–45, 164, 180
Steward, Theolpilus G., 153–55
Stoltz, Paul, 118

terrorism, first use of biological weapons in United States, 187; Native American charges, 188; World War I, 188–90; Geneva Protocol, 190–91; World War II US vaccination program, 193–94; Japanese research on yellow fever, 193–95; German nerve gas, 194–95; anthrax, 209–10; Islamic perspective, 211–15; yellow fever scenario for terrorism, 212–16
Treaty of Paris, 103
trichothecene mycotoxins, 217
Truman, President Harry. S, 197–98
tularemia, 221–22

USS Maine, 151–52

Vicksburg, Mississippi, 114–15, 119–21, 126, 134–35, 138, 256, 265

Wade, Belle, 73–78, 84–86, 91–92; comes down with yellow fever, 94, 96
Warner, Lena, 159, 163
Washington, George, 21–22, 28, 30–32
Washington, Martha, 21–22, 31
West Nile virus, 235
Wharton, Mayor Ramsey, 138
Winchester, James, 64
Winchester, Marcus B., 64
World Health Organization (WHO), on global warming, 230

yellow fever, Japanese research, 193–95, 198; biological weapons, 210–14; vaccinations in the United States, 194–95; symptoms, 243–46, 250; how to protect yourself, 246–47; vaccination, 248–49

Yellow Fever Commission, 184

Yellow Fever National Relief Commission, 92–93